Walking Your Way To Better Health

The 30-day walking to better health compass challenge

Dr. Chio Ugochukwu

Walking Your Way To Better Health

Copyright©2024 Dr. Chio Ugochukwu

All Rights Reserved. No part of this work may be reproduced in any form, or means, without the permission of the author or publisher.

Published by Bundant Enterprises
3053 Rancho Vista Blvd H-197
Palmdale , CA 93551

ISBN: 9798343453409

Printed in the United States of America

Walking Your Way To Better Health

Disclaimer

The information contained in this book is based on research and the personal and professional experience of the author. It is solely for informational and educational purposes and should not be regarded as a substitute for professional, legal, tax, psychological or medical advice. Any attempt to diagnose or treat an illness should be done under the care of a healthcare professional. The author and publisher do not advocate any healthcare protocol but believe the information in this book should be available to the public. Ideas on ways people can get more peace and happiness in their relationships and their lives are shared in this book. The author assumes no liability or responsibility for any adverse effects or consequences from the use of any information, ideas or instruction contained in this book.

Walking Your Way To Better Health

Dedication

The Compass book of 30-day challenges consists of many volumes of books that are dedicated to improving self-mastery, better health, and becoming better versions of ourselves. This Compass book of 30-day challenges vol.3, is the 30-day compass walking to better health challenge for those who want to live a healthier, longer and better life through walking at least 10,000 steps every day. Are you ready to overcome the distractions and doubts that have been stopping you from beginning your own 30-day walking to better health challenge ?

Walking Your Way To Better Health

Table of Content

Walking Your Way To Better Health

Walking Your Way To Better Health

Walking Your Way To Better Health

"Desire is the key to motivation.
But it's determination and commitment to an unrelenting pursuit of your goal....A commitment to excellence...that will enable you to attain the success you seek."

Mario Andretti

Walking Your Way To Better Health

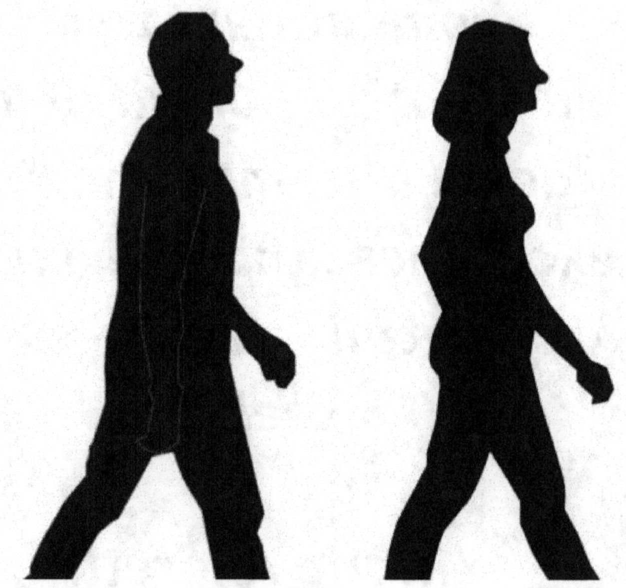

Walking Your Way To Better Health

Introduction

Do you want to stay healthy, active, independent, and live a more fulfilled life as you get older, or do you want to spend your time unintentionally going from one clinic and hospital to another being treated for one illness or another? Take today's challenge and start walking!

After many years of trying different ways of helping myself and others improve their health and wellness and live a healthier, happier and longer life, I found out that doing 30-day challenges is one of the best ways to hold yourself accountable and help you form the purpose-driven holistic habits that will help you achieve specific goals and improve specific aspects of your life one step and one day at a time.

There are different 30-day compass challenges to use to become better at managing daily stress, maintaining a healthy weight, and becoming better at taking care of yourself through more consistent self-care and the challenges that will help you develop holistic habits and simple steps to live a healthier, longer and better life. This Walking Your Way To Better Health is the third volume in the compass book of 30-day challenges.

If you want to be able to hang out with your friends, go on vacations, participate in your friends' milestones or your kids and grandkids milestones like graduations, birthdays, weddings and other festivals and events that you enjoy doing as you get older, then read this book. You will learn how to use the 30-day walking to better health challenge to help you consistently improve your whole-body health.

You will also learn practical and easy ways to make adjustments that will help you improve your self-care and increase your peace of mind and joy of living as you get older. You will learn how to live the telomeric lifestyle! The telomeric lifestyle is the walking lifestyle !

Walking Your Way To Better Health

Did you know that the first key to living a longer and healthier life is consistency in your daily exercise and physical activity? Don't live in denial or form the habit of always having reasons or excuses for not doing your daily exercise. Don't forget that with the help of the compass profile and the compass method the transformation that you need is within your power.

You can use the tips and strategies in the chapters of this book to develop the blueprint that will help you to consistently walk 10,000 steps or more steps a day that will help you walk your way to better health over the next 30 days by doing your own 30-day walking your way to better health challenge!

Walking Your Way To Better Health

Walking Your Way To Better Health

12 COMPASS WALKING YOUR WAY TO BETTER HEALTH GUIDELINES

Do you?	1	2	3	4	5	6	7	8	9	10
Meditate on 3 things you are grateful for daily										
Do 10,000 steps daily										
Sleep At Least 7 hours A Day										
Walk at least 50 minutes every day										
Do daily self-accountability										
Effectively manage daily stress										
Lower daily expectations										
Maintain a healthy weight										
Keep your health vigilance										
Have Supportive relationships										
Eat five servings of vegetables and fruit daily										
Write 3 good things that happened to you every day										

Before you go further in this **Walking Your Way To Better Health Compass 30-day challenge**, begin by doing a self-evaluation on how consistently you use or follow the 12 compass walking your way to better health guidelines for living a healthier and longer life. Mark X on the number that represents how frequently you consistently carry out the compass guidelines in your daily life. You can do this by checking how well you have practiced these guidelines in the past 14 days or 2 weeks or how you will practice them in the next 14 days.

A score of 1 means that you are either practicing a guideline 1 out of 14 days or not at all in your daily life. Mark a score of 2 if you practice or do the guideline only 2 days out of 14 days. Mark a score of 3, if you practice or do the guideline 3 days out of 14 days or every two weeks. A mark of 4 means you are practicing the guideline 4 out of 14 days every two weeks. A mark of 5 means you are practicing or doing the guideline 5 days out of 14 days or every 2 weeks. A mark of 6 means you are practicing or doing the guidelines 6 to 7 days out of 14 days or every two weeks, and a mark of 7, means that you are practicing the guideline 8 to 9 days out 14 days or every 2 weeks. A mark of 8 means that you are practicing the guidelines 10 to 11 days out 14 days or every 2 weeks, a mark of 9 means that you are practicing the guideline 12 to 13 days out 14 days or every 2 weeks. A mark of 14 means that you are practicing the guideline 14 days out 14 days or every 2 weeks.

The more you consistently practice or make use of the guidelines every day the better your health will become. If the total score of the numbers you have marked for all the guidelines is 12, it shows that you are doing each guideline 1 day or not all out of 14 days or every 2 weeks and you are very inconsistent in putting the guidelines into daily practice. A total score of 120 will show that you are very consistent in following the guidelines every day or 14 days out of 14 days, and you are doing a great job.

A total score of 48 or less shows that you have low consistency in practicing your compass guidelines. A score of 49 to less than 96 shows that you have moderate consistency in practicing your own compass guidelines, and a score of 96 to 120 shows high consistency in practicing your own compass guidelines. Most people will have a total score of between 49 and less than 96. You can use your total score to determine which compass guidelines you are more consistently practicing, and which guidelines you need to work on.

Keep a bi-weekly tab on your numbers so that you can hold yourself accountable and help you improve by using the compass profile that I will share with you in this book to gain a deeper insight into yourself together with the compass method for continuous self-improvement or self-mastery to develop your own compass blueprint for becoming a better version of yourself.

Here are the three steps of the compass method you can use to help in walking your way to better health. The first step is doing your own 72-hour audit to find out where you are in your journey of achieving or becoming better at a specific aspect of your life such as walking your way to better health. The first step in applying the compass method to walking your way to better health is to find out how consistently you walk 10,000 steps every day.

The second step is to find out factors that either affect how consistently you walk every day or factors that affect or help you to explain the benefits you will get from walking. These factors could be from yourself, those you interact with, and the space or environment in which you operate.

The third step in the compass method for achieving or becoming better at a specific aspect of your life such as walking your way to better health is to develop a blueprint that would allow you to step by step do the possible based on the factors that you have looked at, the resources that you have, and the sustainable framework that would help walk your way to better health. This will also help you to live in harmony with yourself, your community and your spirit.

You can use the following **compass mantras**, to support your thoughts and actions, diffuse tension and use the ideas and strategies that I will share with you in this book, to achieve the changes you want in your life as you continue to walk your way to better health:

Begin where you are with what you have. It is better to begin with what you have rather than wait for the perfect situation with perfect resources.

Improvement never ends. Focus on improving rather than allowing those who criticize you or point out your failures discourage you from taking daily transformative action.

A mistake is not a failure. It is an opportunity to become better. Everyone makes mistakes but only those with a positive warrior mindset learn from them and focus on how to minimize them and get better results.

Remember that a lapse is not a relapse. Don't beat yourself up if you fail to do 10,000 steps a day. Begin again.

The smallest action is better than the greatest intention. Try to reduce complex steps to small segments that you can accomplish. **Step by step do the possible!**

Remember that to foresee is to rule. This is part of the operational capacity in the compass profile. Anticipating a stressor is the first step towards managing it.

Remember that inadequate preparation leads to failure.

See problems as gifts.

See challenges as opportunities.

See criticisms as tests.

Explanations explain nothing.

Use positive self -talk to counter the negativity from critics.

Lower your expectations from your interactions with others. This will help you lower the gap between what they say or do to you and reduce the stress and frustration you will get from such an interaction.

Hurt begets hurt. When people feel that you have hurt them, they will try to hurt back no matter how you try to explain.

Say crickets when people try to rattle you. Just smile silently inside and focus on becoming better.

Do another self-evaluation at the end of your 30-day challenge for walking your way to better health to find out how your scores have changed and how you have improved or the areas you will need to improve on to get more consistent better health results and benefits as you continue to walk your way to better health.

Begin your walking to better health today by taking 10,000 steps per day

Do an audit of how many steps you have taken in the past 3 days. How many steps on average do you take every day? Do you walk at least 10,000 steps every day? Why is walking daily important? **Research has shown that people as old as 69 years and above who exercise regularly have the heart, lung, and muscle fitness of healthy people as young as 30 years and younger (Crouch, 2019).** Walking is one of the easiest ways you can exercise regularly. What is your motivation for walking 10,000 steps every day? Wouldn't you like to become healthier as you get older or have more stamina as you get older?

Begin your 30-day walking to better health challenge by going for 10,000 steps a day. If you are already used to walking more steps per day, you can set your own goal of 15,000 or 20,000 steps per day. If you have been mostly sedentary and haven't done much walking, begin with 20 minutes of walking or 2,000 steps per day. If you already do 6,000 steps every day, challenge yourself to add another 2,000 steps today. If you already do 10,000 steps a day or about 100 minutes of walking a day, challenge yourself to add another 2,000 steps per day. Research and studies indicate that increasing your physical activity can help you live a healthier and longer life.

If you don't know how many steps you take every day, do your own 72-hour walking audit to determine how many steps you take on average every day. Don't forget that in this 30-day compass walking your way to better health challenge, starting is more important than delaying or procrastinating.

Here are a few things you need to do as part of your 30-day challenge:

Walking Your Way To Better Health

*Walk with what you have or get some comfortable walking shoes. If you are going to do most of your walking inside the house, you can walk barefoot. If you are walking outside the house, in the street or in the park, make sure your environment is safe.

 *Walk 10,000 steps today if you are already used to walking, if not begin with 2,000 steps today or about 20 minutes of walking today.

*Write down how many minutes of exercise you did on day 1. Did you do 15 minutes, 30 minutes, 45 minutes, 60 minutes or 100 minutes that day?

What is the integrative link between exercise and physical activity and antiaging and living longer? **It is the telomere or specific-DNA structures found at both ends of the chromosomes in our cells**. This will help you know the cellular or micro factors that can affect your health.

Walking Your Way To Better Health

According to Bringham Young University researchers, exercise has antiaging effects at the cellular level because increasing physical activity increased the length of telomeres at the end of chromosomes which are usually shorter with age. The study also found that those who exercise had a "biological age" that was about nine years younger(Baines, 2020; Crouch 2019). Why does increasing the length of telomeres in cells have such a positive impact on longevity?

Research shows that those with shorter telomeres have a poorer survival or shorter lifespan, due to an increase in mortality from heart and infectious diseases.

Why is telomere length important? Telomere length is sometimes seen as a biological clock that can be used to determine the lifespan of a cell and an organism (Shammas,2011).

*Do you know that there are many lifestyle changes or factors that can affect the length of your telomere?

Walking Your Way To Better Health

Lack of exercise is one of the lifestyle factors that can significantly shorten your telomere length and could reduce your health and longevity.

*Write down how many hours you spent sitting down today?

Therefore, if you choose to spend most of your time sitting down without exercise, you are choosing a less telomeric lifestyle.

Research also shows that telomere length is more in active people than inactive people, irrespective of whether the exercise was vigorous or moderate. Keeping your telomere length longer for a longer period of time should be one of the reasons that will motivate you to more consistently walk 10,000 steps every day.

How many minutes did you spend exercising or staying physically active today? Write it down.

Remember that 10 minutes of walking is about 1,000 steps. Since on average people have 2 to 2.5 feet per step, it takes about 2,000 steps to cover a mile. This means that

Walking Your Way To Better Health

10,000 steps per day is equal to 100 minutes of exercise every day and about 5 miles of walking every day.

While the main goal of the 30-day walking your way to better health challenge is to get you to walk at least 10,000 steps every day, starting from day 1, one way you can get to its equivalent of 100 minutes of daily physical activity is to begin with 20 minutes of walking which you can combine with the steps from the steps you take during activities like doing your chores, walking from one meeting to another, gardening or during other outdoor activities, to find out the total number of minutes, steps or miles, you have done in a day.

An important integrative link is learning how physical activity affects your cellular and vascular health. As you already know, consistent physical activity helps to increase the length of your telomeres at the cellular level by helping to decrease the rate of shortening of telomeres that occur with age.

What is the impact of exercise at the vascular level? Exercise protects the endothelium or cells lining the vessels by reducing reactive oxygen species and reducing inflammation and increases the cellular metabolic state by affecting your increasing mitochondria (Sorriento, Vaia and Iaccarino, 2021).

Mitochondria are critical to human health and in organs in which damaged mitochondria accumulate more organ damage or disorders occur(Sorriento, Vaia and Iaccarino, 2021).

The integrative strategy here is to think of your mitochondria anytime you exercise or feel like not exercising. You can compare mitochondria to the energy source in your house or the batteries in your computers or smart phones or devices. No matter how expensive your phone is or how well the circuit in your computer is you cannot do much with it when the battery is not working, or the energy source is unreliable or malfunctioning. When the mitochondria or energy packets in your cells malfunction, a lot can go wrong in your mind, body and spirit.

Whenever possible, you should take the stairs instead of the elevator, as little things like that will do wonders for your body. Research has shown that if you started exercising between 40 and 60 years of age, you would reduce your risk of having stroke that can significantly reduce your chances of living longer. This shows that it is really never too late to start exercising or form the habit of consistently increasing the level of your physical activity.

Do not think that it is either you are getting everything right or everything is wrong. Remember that one of the mantras in the compass method, is step by step do the possible. If you plan to walk 60 minutes a day but due to circumstances beyond your control you were able to do only 25 minutes, you have not failed. Do the 25 minutes that day, then do 95 minutes the next day to make it up. This still makes a total of 120 minutes in two days. On the third day you can go back to 60 minutes a day. Be flexible.

Make sure you keep track of your progress. Fill tables 1A and 1B in the next pages to track your progress. Write down the number of steps you take every day, number of minutes of walking, and the reason for walking, and the reasons for not walking. Tracking how well you are doing is part of the second step in the compass method because it will help you discover the factors that affect how well you are doing. Writing down a comment will help keep track of your positive, negative and neutral days. What will you do differently on the negative days? How many steps do you take every day? Remember that the goal is to make walking every day a new holistic habit that works for you in the context of your situation and circumstances.

Walking Your Way To Better Health

TABLE 1A

Day	Number Of Steps	Minutes of walking	Motivation For walking	Reason For Not Walking	comment
1					
2					
3					
4					
5					
6					
7					
8					
9					
10					
11					
12					
13					
14					
15					

Walking Your Way To Better Health

TABLE 1B

Day	Number Of Steps	Minutes of walking	Motivation For walking	Reason For Not Walking	comment
16					
17					
18					
19					
20					
21					
22					
23					
24					
25					
26					
27					
28					
29					
30					

Walking Your Way To Better Health

Do you consistently walk 10,000 steps every day or do you get distracted?

What are the distractions stopping you from being consistent with your daily 10,000 steps? Were you distracted or too tired to get to 10,000 steps on day1? Try again on day 2 or day 3.

What distracted you?

Was it watching TV?

Was it talking on the phone?

Was it playing too much on your phone or device or computer?

Was it always putting off, when you would actually begin to walk?

Was it a negative encounter or interaction?

Focus on what you can control is a compass mantra. Remember that distractions get the better of you, when you do not focus on what you can control. Be intentional. Spend time doing the things that would help you become better and stop wasting time on things that only give momentary pleasure without adding value to your life.

Don't let distractions stop you from consistent physical activity. Remember that research shows that exercise can help you boost your mood, help you sleep better, help you keep a healthy weight, improve your immune system, digestive function, and your brain health, in addition to its impact on the length of your telomere which can help you to slow down on aging and help you live a longer life.

Fill out Tables 2A and 2B and write down the number of distractions you had per day based on how you answered the questions on possible distractions or your own experience. When you track what you are doing, you put yourself in a better position to form the holistic habits that will help you improve.

Remind yourself of why you are doing this 30-day compass walking your way to better health challenge. You want to stay healthy so that so spend quality time with yourself, your family and your friends as you get older.

Is your mood one of the distractions that could prevent you from having more consistent physical activity?

How can you walk more consistently? You can do this by setting daily objectives and the actions you can take to achieve those objectives. You can begin by finding simple but consistent ways to walk for about 30 minutes every day. If you don't have 30 minutes in one block, break up your exercise into 10 or 15 minutes each. Remember that 10 minutes of walking is about 1,000 steps. Since on average people have 2 to 2.5 feet per step, it takes about 2,000 steps to cover a mile. This means that 10,000 steps a day is about 5 miles a day

Did you know that if you keep on putting off when you exercise, you may end up not doing it? My father in-law used to say that "Procrastination is the thief of time".

Don't procrastinate, do your exercise first in the morning or simply get up and do your exercise once the thought crosses your mind.

When you fill tables 2A and 2 B below, note how many days you failed to walk 10,000 steps , and how many distractions you had that day. How will you overcome such distractions in the next 7 days, and in the next 30 days? Remember that the key to getting the most health benefits from walking is consistency.

TABLE 2A

Day	Number Of Steps	Minutes of walking	Number of distractions
1			
2			
3			
4			
5			
6			
7			
8			
9			
10			
11			
12			
13			
14			
15			

TABLE 2B

Day	Number Of Steps	Minutes of walking	Number of distractions
16			
17			
18			
19			
20			
21			
22			
23			
24			
25			
26			
27			
28			
29			
30			

Set the goal of maintaining a healthy weight by losing one to two pounds every one to two weeks by walking

Specificity leads to focus. Remember that you need to set simple goals that you have the means to accomplish. This is part of the operational capacity of the compass profile. This is why on day 3 of your 30-day walking your way to better health challenge, I want you to set the specific goal of losing at least one and a quarter pounds per week through walking.

How can you do this?

First weigh yourself .

Second, write the number of steps you take every day so that you will know what adjustments you need to make to help you lose one to two pounds every two weeks.

Walking Your Way To Better Health

If you want to lose 5 pounds in one month, it means you want to lose 2.5 pounds in 2 weeks, leading to 5 pounds in 4 weeks. You can lose 5 pounds in a month without changing much about what you eat by simply increasing the number of steps you take every day. If you used to walk only 5,000 steps a day, can you lose 2.5 pounds in a week? The answer would be No, because 5,000 steps a day would lead to losing 250 calories per day and five hundred calories in 2 days.

Since research shows that 3,500 calories of energy equal 1 pound, you would burn off 3,500 to lose 1 pound. If you are walking 5,000 steps a day, it will take you 14 days to lose 1 pound, if you keep to your usual eating pattern. If you want to lose weight by eating less than 3,500 calories per day, it would be impossible or starvation since we need about 2,000 to 2,500 calories of energy for our usual daily activities.

A more practical approach to maintaining a healthy weight would be eating a little less every day and walking more steps every day. A less drastic and more sustainable approach would be to walk 10,000 steps per day so that you can burn off or lose 500 calories per day, leading to burning off about 3,500 calories per week or losing one pound per week by walking 70,000 steps per week. If you decide to do 20,000 steps per day, you would be walking 140,000 steps per week and would be losing about 2 pounds per week.

While you can possibly lose one pound per week by walking 10,000 steps per day, if you find that your schedule makes this difficult, don't be discouraged. You can begin with doing 5,000 steps per day, which would lead to 35,000 steps per week or 70,000 steps in 2 weeks or burning off 3,500 calories in 2 weeks or losing one pound in 2 weeks.

Don't try to do all these calculations, just use a pedometer to track how many steps you are taking every day or every week. To lose one to two pounds in one to two weeks, you need to consistently walk 5,000 to 10,000 steps a day so that you can burn off about 250 calories to 500 calories per day. This is a simple sustainable way of losing about one to 2 pounds in 1 to 2 weeks.

Do you think you can walk 10,000 steps per day? It takes about 10 minutes to walk 1,000 steps, it means it will take about 100 minutes a day to walk 10,000 steps a day. Can you do it? You can break your walks per day into 30 minutes or 10 to 15 minutes walk. A more realistic way of meeting your goal of regular physical activity for you might be to begin by finding simple but consistent ways to walk for about 30 minutes every day. If you don't have 30 minutes in one block, break up your exercise into 10 or 15 minutes each. Remember that 10 minutes of walking is about 1,000 steps. Since on average people have 2 to 2.5 feet per step, it takes about 2,000 steps to cover a mile. This means that 10,000 steps a day is about 5 miles a day.

The good news is that you can combine the steps from your formal physical activity period with the steps you take during activities like doing your chores, walking from one meeting to another, gardening or during other outdoor activities, to find out the total number of minutes, steps or miles, you have done in a day.

When you are trying to walk yourself to better health continue to add at least 500 more steps per day, until you get to an average of 10,000 steps per day. If you are not getting to 10,000 steps per day, look at daily comments to see the adjustments you need to make. When you are more consistent with at least 10,000 steps per day, you can take it to the next level by doing 20.000 steps per day.

Walking Your Way To Better Health

Use walking to meet a realistic goal of at least 50 minutes of daily physical activity

How many minutes of physical activity do you need every week? Keep in mind that the minimum moderate intensity physical activity such as walking, that was recommended by the WHO and the CDC for better health, is about 150 minutes per week or at least 30 minutes per day for 5 days in a week.

Doing at least 50 minutes of daily physical activity is one of the easiest ways to meet the minimum requirement of 30 minutes a day as recommended by the WHO and CDC and achieve better health. Do you now consistently walk at least 10,000 steps a day? If you are walking at least 10,000 steps per day, then you are doing about 100 minutes of physical activity per day. Is this a realistic goal for you or do you want to set a goal of about 5,000 steps a day to begin with? Even if you are able to walk only 5,000 steps, you are doing at least 50 minutes of physical activity per day.

How many minutes of physical activities did you do today? Most guidelines recommend about 150 minutes per week of moderate physical activity. What does 150 minutes of exercise per week mean? I already explained that it means you are doing about 30 minutes of exercise per day for at least 5 days a week.

Do you know that according to the National Institute of Health, only about 30 percent of people between 45 years and 64 years engage in leisure-time physical activity, and for those 65 years above the percentage drops to 15 percent and less (NIH News, 2017). According to the AARP, only about 17 % of Americans 50 years and above, do at least 150 minutes of exercise every week.

Walking Your Way To Better Health

If your main exercise is walking, it means you are taking about 3000 steps per day since 1000 steps is equal to about 10 minutes of physical activity. Why is increasing your daily physical activity(PA) such an important part of making yourself healthier and living longer as you get older?

Research shows that a sedentary lifestyle is considered a significant risk factor for cardiovascular disease while consistently doing more physical activity could be considered a non-pharmacological intervention for improving cardiovascular fitness in healthy and diseased individuals.

Your goal at the end of your 30-day walking your way to better health challenge should be walking at least 10,000 steps per day. On day one, find out the steps you walked. You can measure your steps per day with a pedometer or with a smart watch and get your average for the first 7 days then challenge yourself to meet up your goal by adding to your average in the next 7 days.

Walking Your Way To Better Health

How will your realistic goals motivate you? They are achievable goals that can encourage you to become more active.

Don't allow daily distractions to prevent you from meeting your daily physical activity goals. Always strive to live a positive and fulfilled life.

Make sure you track your progress by filling tables 3 A and 3B. You can even challenge yourself to walk at least 200 minutes every day. Keep in mind your operational capacity and your ambition profile. Use the resources you have to make sure your goals are realistic and achievable. Step by step do the possible.

Here are some of the motivations that people may have for wanting to walk many steps every day:

Better shape
More relaxation
Better sleep
Improved movement
Less painful joints

Walking Your Way To Better Health

Better health
Better eye health
Better heart health
Better brain health
Living longer

What would you do if you were not able to get to 10,000 steps per day at the end of the first 30-day challenge? Begin another 30 - day challenge specifically for walking and try to do 5,000 steps in the first week, then 10,000 steps a day from the 2nd to the week, 4th week of your 30-day walking your way to better health challenge.

Walking Your Way To Better Health

TABLE 3 A

Day	Number Of Steps	Minutes of walking	Motivation For walking	How many distractions did you overcome	comment
1					
2					
3					
4					
5					
6					
7					
8					
9					
10					
11					
12					
13					
14					
15					

Walking Your Way To Better Health

TABLE 3 B

Day	Number Of Steps	Minutes of walking	Motivation For walking	How many distractions did you overcome	comment
16					
17					
18					
19					
20					
21					
22					
23					
24					
25					
26					
27					
28					
29					
30					

Did you know that walking many steps a day can help you sleep better and have better health?

How many hours of sleep did you have today? Was it 5 hours of sleep, 6 hours , 7 hours or 8 hours?

*Write down how many hours of sleep you had on day 5. You can also write it down in your health and wellness journal or in your device or the journal part of this book that you are using for doing your own 30-day walking your way to better health challenge.

Do you know why the number of hours you sleep every day can affect how long and healthy you will live? According to the CDC, 1 out of 3 adults do not get enough sleep or about 7 hours of sleep every night (CDC, 2016). According to the American Academy of Sleep Medicine and the Sleep

Research Society, adults aged 18 to 60, need about 7 hours of sleep every night for great health and well-being. Sleeping less than 7 hours every night predisposes one to more chronic conditions like heart disease, diabetes, stroke, mental stress or depression, and obesity. This is consistent with the research that shows that there is an association between chronic poor sleep quality and an increased risk for age-related disease, mental health deterioration, and dying early (Sabot, Lovegrove, and Stapleton, 2023).

Do you know why having poor sleep predisposes one to poor health?

Here is an important integrative link you can use for your own compass blueprint for living a longer and better life. Research shows that inadequate sleep is associated with cellular damage through negative effects on telomere length (Sabot, Lovegrove, and Stapleton, 2023). Research also shows that sleep helps restore the body's nervous, immune, muscular, and skeletal systems. This restorative process is crucial for cognitive functions, such as emotional regulation and memory, and overall health and well-being (Sabot, Lovegrove, and Stapleton, 2023). The other thing to remember is that poor sleep includes the number of hours you have slept, how long it takes you to fall asleep and whether you wake up feeling rested or not.

Remember that the more you increase the amount of physical exercise that you participate in during the day, the easier it will be for you to sleep well. This is one of the ways to help you get a good sleep at night. The more active your body is during the day, the more likely you are to relax at night and fall asleep faster.

If you doubt this, watch your children. You will find out that they sleep the most when they have been most busy running around and actively playing all day. They get into bed and fall sound asleep.

Walk to good health by walking many steps every day. You'll notice that your quality of sleep is improved and the transition between the cycles and phases of sleep will become smoother and more regular. By keeping up your physical activity during the day, you may find it easier to deal with the stress and worries of your life.

*Write down how many steps you walked today. Did you walk at least 12,000 steps today? How many hours of sleep did you have today? The goal is to have 7 or more hours of sleep every day.

During this 30-day compass walking your way to better health challenge your goal is to increase the number of steps you take every day, reduce the number of hours you spend on TV and devices, and cut down disruptions like arguing, eating late or working late that make you sleep for fewer hours. Please fill out tables 3A and 3B, so that you can learn more about your sleeping pattern and the adjustments you need to make to sleep more.

Walking Your Way To Better Health

TABLE 4A

Day	Number Of Steps	Hours on TV	Number of Distractions	Hours of Sleep
1				
2				
3				
4				
5				
6				
7				
8				
9				
10				
11				
12				
13				
14				
15				

Walking Your Way To Better Health

TABLE 4B

Day	Number Of Steps	Hours on TV	Number of Distractions	Hours of Sleep
16				
17				
18				
19				
20				
21				
22				
23				
24				
25				
26				
27				
28				
29				
30				

Pay attention to how walking many steps every day can affect your blood pressure and your numbers

Are you healthy or do you simply feel healthy without truly knowing if you are healthy or not? Do you know your blood pressure? **Do you know your numbers?** Knowing your numbers is part of the Compass metabolic and physical profiles.

Please write down your weight, height and BMI. If you don't know your numbers or have not had a physical this year, please see your doctor and have one. When was the last time you checked your blood pressure or went for a physical?

Even if you had previously weighed yourself or day 2, weigh yourself again on day 8.

Write down your weight and waist circumference. If you are feeling healthy but you don't know your blood pressure, how do you know that you are healthy.

Do you know if your blood pressure is 110/70mmHg or 130/80mmHg or 200/110mmHg? High blood pressure is one the most common chronic conditions that can affect your health and longevity?

The previous guidelines considered a blood pressure of 140/90 mmHg to be high blood pressure but since 2017 the new AHA guidelines defined high blood pressure as a reading of 130/80 mmHg and anything between 120 to 129 mm Hg as elevated.

If your blood pressure is 190/100mmHg and you didn't know it, you're a ticking time bomb for a major life altering or possibly life-ending event like a stroke or heart attack. A few years ago, a 53-year-old man, who was in apparent good health or felt healthy collapsed and died after a failed resuscitation. Before he died, EMT found out that his blood pressure was 260/150 mmHg , and he had had a heart attack while exercising. His wife, who was with him in the gym when he collapsed, said he had always been in relatively good health and was not on any medications.

This example of someone dying while exercising is important because too many people think that simply because they exercise regularly, eat healthy, sleep well and have no symptoms, then they must be in good health. If you ask them about their blood pressure or weight, they won't know. They will tell you they don't need to do anything or worry because they are doing well and do not need to do anything else. This is a wrong and potentially deadly assumption. High blood pressure is a silent killer, you could have it without having symptoms.

You need to know your own numbers. You need to have an idea of the potential illnesses you could be dealing with as you get older based on your family history, past medical history and age group. Do you know your family history? Do you have diabetes, high blood pressure or kidney disease in your family? Do you know the commonest cause of illness or death in your age group as you get older? If you want to live longer, it is important that you pay attention to what has happened to others or is happening to most people your age.

For this challenge, all you need to do is to measure your blood pressure every day for the next 30 days and make comments about whether you did or did not. Fill Tables 5A and 5B. In the comments write down if you slept well or not, write down how many hours you slept, what was your compass stress index for the day, and did you eat five servings of fruits and vegetables? If you have not yet done your yearly physical or gone for your yearly check up with your primary care provider, do it.

Walking Your Way To Better Health

TABLE 5A

Day	Blood Pressure	weight	Number of daily steps	Comments
1				
2				
3				
4				
5				
6				
7				
8				
9				
10				
11				
12				
13				
14				
15				

Walking Your Way To Better Health

TABLE 5B

Day	Blood Pressure	weight	Number of daily steps	Comments
16				
17				
18				
19				
20				
21				
22				
23				
24				
25				
26				
27				
28				
29				
30				

Make sure you are managing the leading causes of death for your age group

Please, don't make the mistake of assuming that because you are walking every day, you must be so healthy that you don't have to see your doctor. Don't assume that because you are not on any medications, and you don't have any symptoms of illness, and you haven't been to the doctor in years and are feeling well, then you must be healthy. This is not always true. If you don't have concrete data and verified medical opinion telling you that your health status is good, don't assume you have optimal health.

How many times have you heard about someone who was healthy and working out regularly and was full of life, who suddenly slumped and died? How many times did the news report also state that the person had high blood pressure but didn't know? One way to help yourself minimize the risk of such an experience is to begin your own journey towards using integrative strategies and simple habits and ways to have a more consistent healthy lifestyle.

Worldwide leading causes of death for older people are the following:

Heart disease
Stroke
COPD
Lower respiratory infections.

You need to pay attention to the common causes of death and illness for your age group. According to the National Council on Aging (NCOA) the leading causes of death among older people in the US are heart disease, cancer, C0VID-19, stroke, chronic lower respiratory diseases, Alzheimer's, and diabetes (NCOA,2023).

US leading causes of death for older people are the following:

Heart disease
Cancer
COVID-19
Stroke
Chronic lower respiratory diseases
Alzheimer's
Diabetes

The interesting thing about this is that 5 years ago or in 2018, it would not have included COVID 19. This shows one of the reasons why everyone must remain vigilant. Things change, and we have to learn to take notice and make our own adjustments.

According to the WHO, the leading causes of death among older people, worldwide are **heart disease, stroke, chronic obstructive pulmonary disease, and lower respiratory infections (WHO, 2020).** We need to keep these leading causes of death or illness in mind when making our own health and wellness decisions and actions.

How can you make sure you are managing the leading causes of death for your age group? Go and see your doctor and get your labs done. Write down your blood pressure and weight. Make a note of what part of your family history or even your medical history you need to pay particular attention to.

*Write down your blood sugar or find out your blood sugar level.
*Do you smoke? You need to stop smoking.
*How many cigarettes did you smoke today?
*How much alcohol did you drink today?

If you have not yet done a medical or health checkup or physical in years and you have no idea what your blood pressure is or what your weight, blood sugar or cholesterol level, then your physical.

Have you done your age-related screening tests like your PSA or colonoscopy?

Go and see your doctor and get some labs done to get a data-based health assessment of your health status. Do you know your blood sugar level? Do you know your cholesterol level? How well are your kidneys and liver functioning?

Let's face it! Most of us think we are very healthy. This is a common thought for young adults and middle-aged adults. Yet we all know that looks can be deceiving. I am sure you have all heard stories of people who were apparently very healthy then suddenly died from a heart attack or cancer after a "brief illness" or even had a near death experience (NDE).

The most important thing to remember is that while walking 10,000 steps can help you live a healthier and happier life, you still need to see your doctor and follow up on the common causes of death for your age group and get your blood work done. How well have you been managing the leading causes of death for your group? Challenge yourself to do your labs in the next 14 days while still doing your 10,000 steps per day.

Walking Your Way To Better Health

Walking can help you lower your LDL, increase your HDL, and improve your heart health

Do you know that walking is one of the natural ways you can improve your heart health? What do you need to know? You need to know that heart disease is among the leading causes of death for middle-aged men and women in most parts of the world, including the United States and Western Europe. Even in developing countries like Nigeria the trend toward more deaths related to heart disease is becoming more common.

Have you measured your blood pressure in the past 7 days? As part of your walking to better health strategy you should measure your blood pressure regularly . If possible do it daily. If you haven't, measure it today and measure it every other day or as directed by your doctor. Start your own blood

---

pressure log or review the 72-hour health and wellness audit that you did before.

Do you have any friends that suddenly had a stroke or died from heart attack?

Do you have any friends, relatives, colleagues, or siblings that unexpectedly had heart attacks and survived? This what I typically call a near death experience (NDE).

Do you want to have your own NDE, before you begin to take the steps that will help you to reduce your cardiovascular risk factors and improve your own heart health?

Walking is one of the easiest ways you can reduce your cardiovascular risk factors.

The factors that can affect your heart health include the following:

Age
Sex
Weight
Blood pressure

Walking Your Way To Better Health

Blood sugar
Smoking
Drinking alcohol
Family History
Triglyceride Level
HDL or good cholesterol
LDL or bad cholesterol

High blood pressure, stroke and heart attack and other related heart diseases are common problems that you could experience as you get older. What are you going to do about them?

*Do you know your blood pressure today?

Some of the ways you can reduce your blood pressure or keep it at about 120/80 mmHg will be to first measure it, watch what you eat, cut down on your sodium intake, manage stress better, exercise more, and live more of a telomeric lifestyle.

*Weigh yourself and write down your weight today. This is an example of how knowing your numbers can affect different aspects of your health. Walking is one of the ways you can maintain a healthy weight and reduce your chances of having a heart attack or other types of heart disease.

You can reduce your risk of having heart disease and other related near death experience (NDE) by reducing your LDL level and increasing your HDL. Getting more details about your lipid-profile and other blood work is part of the compass metabolic profile, which is the fifth component of the compass profiles.

*Write down the last time you saw your doctor or did your blood work? Do you know your lipid profile? Do you know your cholesterol level? If you don't know your cholesterol and you are 40 and above you are making a big mistake, because some health associations recommend that people should start doing a check of their cholesterol level from 20 years of age. Knowing your lipid profile is important because you can use it in computing your cardiovascular risk. Your lipid profile includes your triglyceride level, total cholesterol, HDL (High Density

Walking Your Way To Better Health

Lipoprotein) or good cholesterol, and LDL (Low density Lipoprotein) or bad cholesterol.

You can increase your daily physical activity to at least 50 minutes per day. Walking at least 10,000 steps a day is even better. Increase in daily physical activity improves quality of life, reduces body weight, reduces LDL cholesterol, increases HDL cholesterol, increases insulin sensitivity, and helps to prevent pathologic conditions like obesity, atherosclerosis, diabetes, and decreases blood pressure both at rest and during exercise, thus helping to prevent metabolic syndrome and a hypertensive state (Sorriento, Vaia and Iaccarino, 2021)

What are the benefits of reducing your LDL or bad cholesterol level? According to the CDC, too much LDL can build up in our blood vessels and lead to the buildup of plaque which can increase the risk of heart disease and stroke. This means that high levels of LDL can affect your vascular health. One of the benefits of cutting down LDL is the reduced risk that follows.

In this walking your way to better health challenge, the focus will be on asking yourself if you are regularly doing those things that will help you to lower your LDL, reduce your total triglycerides and increase your HDL.

What is the benefit of having high HDL? According to CDC, HDL or high-density lipoprotein helps to move cholesterol from the blood to the liver. This means a higher level of HDL would help to reduce the risk of heart disease and stroke. Some of the ways you can increase your HDL is through increasing physical activity or exercise.

Make sure you consistently do physical activity that will help lower bad cholesterol and increase good cholesterol. Make sure that you do your labs and lipide profile through your doctor. How consistently are you keeping to walking 10,000 steps every day? What distractions are making it hard for you to be consistent?

Walking Your Way To Better Health

TABLE 6A

Day	Number Of Steps	weight	Blood pressure	Number of out bursts of stress
1				
2				
3				
4				
5				
6				
7				
8				
9				
10				
11				
12				
13				
14				
15				

Walking Your Way To Better Health

TABLE 6B

Day	Number Of Steps	weight	Blood Pressure	Number of out bursts of stress
16				
17				
18				
19				
20				
21				
22				
23				
24				
25				
26				
27				
28				
29				
30				

Walking Your Way To Better Health

You can calculate your own personal risk of having a heart attack by visiting http://hp2010.nhlbihin.net/atpiii/calculator.a sp or simply using the following calculators:

<u>Framingham Risk Calculator (omnicalculator.com)</u>

<u>2018 Prevention Guidelines Tool CV Risk Calculator (heart.org)</u>

The 30-day walking your way to better health challenge is one of the ways you can start working on lowering your cardiovascular risk factor. How many steps did you take today?

Walking daily can help you to maintain a healthy weight

Do you weigh yourself every week? If you weigh yourself daily or at least once every week, it will help you keep your weight healthy by keeping better track of your weight or changes to your weight. This way you can catch negative trends early and begin to make changes early. How many steps do you walk in a week ? Did you take 10,000 steps a day?

Weigh yourself before you start then weigh yourself after every week. You can use a simple scale to weigh yourself. Measuring your weight regularly is one of the easiest checks on how your individualized health plan is working. It is easier to do than calculating your BMI. Just climb on a scale and read your weight.

Walking Your Way To Better Health

Get a weight-loss journal or notebook. Unless you have a way to regularly evaluate your progress throughout your health and wellness loss journey, you will find sustainable success more difficult to maintain. How can you tell if you are meeting your daily mini goals if you don't evaluate yourself? Evaluating yourself regularly and taking daily positive action will help you form the right healthy habits.

While walking daily can help you to lose weight and maintain a healthy weight, it cannot happen in a vacuum. The more you know about how unhealthy food choices can affect your weight, cellular and vascular health, the more you will be interested in making sustainable lifestyle changes. Do you regularly eat your variety vegetables and fruits? If you truly want to maintain a healthy weight you have to combine walking regularly with eating more plant-based food.

Walking Your Way To Better Health

SIMPLE WEIGHT TRACKER

DATE	TIME	WEIGHT	NOTES / COMMENTS

Walking Your Way To Better Health

Do you still exercise regularly or have discovered that "you don't have time"? Are you becoming better at managing stress that could arise out of your interactions, conversations, and relationships with yourself and others?

To lose weight and keep it off track yourself to show whether what you are doing is working or not. You can do this by doing two simple things once a week. Weigh yourself at least once a week and calculate your BMI every three months. Measure your waist circumference once a week. You can also use less formal ways like dress size, change in belt hole, pant size, loose ring, or changes in shoe fitting to evaluate your weight loss journey. Take time to fill in your compass healthy living logbook or journal every day or at least once a week.

This will give you an idea of some factors contributing to your weight gain or stubborn weight loss. Maybe you are not doing enough steps every day and are simply spending too much time watching TV or on social media. According to Cleland,

Schmidt, Dwyer, &Venn, the (2008) time spent in behaviors that involve a lot of sitting with little activity, like watching or viewing TV was thought to be one of the factors responsible for increasing number of people that are either overweight or obese in different parts of the world. The study also found that in both men and women the average time spent watching television increased with the increasing frequency of consuming food and drinks while watching television. Soft drink consumption during television viewing was associated with a greater increase in abdominal obesity in both men and women.

If on the other hand you discover that you have gained back some of the weight you have lost even after a certain number of steps consistently then do a quick 72 –hour food audit to see the eating patterns that are making you gain weight. Short-term weight gains usually are as a result of increasing calorie intake or eating more food, rather than simply from reducing physical activity.

Remember that a lapse is not a relapse. A mistake is not a failure. Don't be too harsh on yourself ! If you find yourself not sticking to the 10,000 steps a day as you had planned, get up and begin again. It is better to keep on trying than to give up because you failed a few times.

What do you say to yourself when you are walking or dealing with daily challenges? Do you know that the kind of self-talk you give yourself can affect your weight? This is part of the process of autosuggestion with which you can direct your subconscious mind. If you tell yourself that you can't lose weight, then you will find a way to gain weight even after you have started losing weight or started making the right adjustments. Try again if you do not succeed the first time.

Do not forget to talk to your doctor or health care provider about your medications. Make sure you are not taking any medications or have any underlying disorders that may make you gain weight. This is particularly important if through a chart of your weekly weight measurement you discover that you have gained weight.

Check your list of activities you consider realistic for you to accomplish your weight loss in a day based on your knowledge, experience, personality, available resources, and your stress management skills. Once you have a concrete list in front of you, it's a lot easier to check on yourself regularly and know what lifestyle changes you will need to make.

Remember that maintaining a healthy weight is part of the telomeric lifestyle. Weigh yourself and calculate your BMI. If you can't do it, see your doctor or provider. A combination of exercise, eating healthy and managing stress with good self-care will help lose weight in a realistic and sustainable way.

Remember to weigh yourself today. Make sure you weigh yourself at least every 3 days, in this compass 30-day walking to better health challenge. It is a way of keeping track of your challenges or progress. You can use tables 6A and 6B to also keep track of the number of steps you take every day and your weight.

Use daily walking to help you effectively manage stress every day

When it comes to managing stress everyday you have to remember that any one of your daily interactions can become a stressor because it can alter the balance or homeostasis within your body system. After all, stress can be defined as a threat to your homeostasis or inner balance caused by a variety of stressors, such as environmental, psychological, or physiological factors (Chung, 2005).

Why is managing stress important for living a healthier and longer life?

Research shows that stress increases the risk of diabetes mellitus, can lead to a buildup of plaque in arteries(atherosclerosis), especially if combined with unhealthy eating and a sedentary lifestyle, and can lead to anxiety, depression, and severe broncho-constriction in asthmatics (Salleh, 2008).

What is the link between walking and your microvascular health? Research has shown that walking helps boost your mood because it increases blood flow and blood circulation to the brain and body. Researchers at New Mexico Highlands University (NMHU) found that the foot's impact during walking sends pressure waves through the arteries that significantly modify and can increase the supply of blood to the brain. Please don't say that you are too stressed out to walk. Walking will help you melt away stress and keep your organs younger! By making sure that you walk at least 10,000 steps every day, you prevent yourself from living a sedentary lifestyle which can lead to a more damaging impact of stress on your cellular and vascular health.

Stress also affects cellular and vascular health by causing increased mitochondrial activity and increased damaging and shortening of.   telomeres. Damaged and shortened telomeres are associated with chronic inflammation and age-related degenerative diseases(Lin and Epel, 2022).

Why should you care about the effect of stress on the length of telomeres? Research found that those 60 years and above with shorter telomere length had earlier all-cause mortality from infectious disease and heart disease (Lin and Epel, 2022).

Stress can affect cellular health by leading to damage to your mitochondria and repeated acute stress in our cells can lead to degenerative diseases, cardiovascular diseases, malignancies, and contribute to the process of aging (Poljšak and Milisav, 2012 ; Chung, 2005).

Research also shows that emotional stress contributes significantly to cancer, cardiovascular disease, accidental injuries, respiratory disorders, liver cirrhosis, and suicide, which are among the leading causes of death in the United States (Salleh,2008). Are you mentally focused enough to maintain your peace of mind and protect your health every day? Walking at 10,000 steps every day will help you build up the positive mood that will help you to more effectively deal with emotional stress.

You also need to do your do your own 72-hour stress audit so that you can find the most common stressors you have to deal with. You can do this by simply writing down the situations and circumstances that led to stress for you in the past 72 hours.

Write down the common causes of stress in your life based on the audit you did. Were they conversational or non-conversational stressors? How can you stay calm under pressure?

How do you deal with stress that comes from your relationship and interactions with others? Is someone close to you always telling you that you are not smart enough? Is someone telling you that you are too lazy to walk 10,000 steps a day?

Do you believe them?

Walking Your Way To Better Health

The best way to manage stress from your relationships is to manage your expectations. Lower your expectations in terms of being treated fairly, being understood or appreciated.

How do you deal with daily hassles such as arguments at work, at home, or at events, annoying drivers, marital problems, financial difficulties, and challenges at work which could be sources of repeated acute stress or sources of chronic stress? Remember that walking increases blood flow to your brain!

Focus on what you can control and don't forget the integrative link between your mind, body, and spirit. You can use mind over matter to manage stress. **According to Marcus Aurelius, "A real man doesn't give way to anger and discontent, ….. The nearer a man can come to a calm mind, the closer he is to strength."**

Learn to look at your conversations with others as a chess game. Don't just talk to others without being mentally prepared for how they would respond to you. This could be a negative response from a person that sees problems in everything you do. With others, it could be a positive response. Remember that if you want to win a chess game, you must be able to anticipate 2 or 3 moves your opponent might make after you have made your first move. When you are talking to others, you must form the habit of anticipating 2 or 3 responses ahead.

In addition to managing conversational stress, do you also manage non-conversational stress. **You can manage non-conversational stress by doing the following:**

- Lower expectations
- Check strategic outcomes/ possibilities
- Step by step do the possible based on your resources, context and time
- Use positive self-talk to help yourself while moving from where you are to where you want to be.
- Make out time to walk more consistently so that you can put

yourself in the positive mood that can help you deal with stress better

How consistently have you anticipated your responses to others in the past 7 days? In the next 30 days write down the circumstances that led to the most challenging encounters you had with others.

Walking can help you manage stress by helping you to lift your mood and clear your head. How manty times do you get into stressful outbursts to the level of losing it in a day? You can simply use the number of stressful outbursts or the compass stress index(CSI) to track how well your daily steps are helping you to manage stress.

If you get into stressful outbursts 10 or more times a week , then your compass stress index is 100 . When it is 5 to 9 times a week, your compass stress index is 50 to 90. When it is 2 to 4 times per week, Your Compass Stress Index will be 20 to 40. When your stressful outburst is 0 or once per week, your CSI will be 0 or 10.

Walking Your Way To Better Health

Your daily objective would be to keep your Compass Stress Index (CSI) to zero per day or one per week, giving a CSI of not more than 10 per week. This means having 1 or less stressful challenging event per week should be your goal.

Here is your modified compass stress index(CSI):

Good Compass stress index: 0 to 1 stress outburst per week

Mild Compass stress index: 2 to 4 stress outbursts per week

Moderate Compass stress index:5 to 9 stress outbursts per week (examples include lashing out at others, cutting others off, insisting on your point of view)

Severe Compass stress index: 10 or more stress outbursts per week (This will include pointing at others, speaking with raised voices or being in people's personal space without touching them)

Extreme Compass stress index: Any compass stress index with any hostile contact.

A compass stress outburst is characterized by non-contact emotional disruption that includes anger, confusion, more silence than usual, yelling, disruptive behavior like tension muscles, pounding or striking things without contact with another person.

Hostile contact with another person in terms of angrily touching others, shoving, pushing, fighting, or using or brandishing weapons like knives, guns, sticks, stones, glass, regardless of frequency of daily stressful outbursts is an automatic extreme compass stress index that would require immediate action to diffuse the tension and protect your life.

Why? **Extreme compass stress index means DANGER.** What actions will you take when your house is on fire? Get out of the house as fast as you can and as safely as you can. Do the same when you are dealing or interacting with someone whose behavior has been classified or found to be dangerous or extreme compass stress index. Get yourself out of the situation or get yourself out of their way. Stay vigilant. **Even the most beautiful butterfly still gets eaten by a bird!**

Write down your average compass stress index for the week and the average number of steps you took for the week. You should strive for a weekly compass stress index of 10 or less or preferably a daily CSI of zero. What is your daily CSI? Review it after week to your trend. Is it going up or going down?

Get a stress-free -living journal or notebook and take notes of the time and circumstances that typically lead to a stressful outburst. This will help you discover your own tendencies, patterns, and the commonest causes of stress for you.

Don't let regular evaluation discourage you, instead use it as a tool to discover either new sources   of   emotional   tension   or   new wrinkles to old sources of emotional tension, so that you can more effectively manage them and protect your health, sense of well-being and happiness.

How is your 30-day walking your way to better challenge going for you? Write down the most common factors or situations that caused you stress in the past 7 days. How many steps did you take on such days and did walking more help you? What is your compass stress index(CSI)? Did you reduce your CSI by at least 80% at the end of the 30-day challenge?

TABLE 7A

Day	Number Of Steps	Compass Stress index (CSI)	comments
1			
2			
3			
4			
5			
6			
7			
8			
9			
10			
11			
12			
13			
14			
15			

TABLE 7B

Day	Number Of Steps	Compass Stress Index(CSI)	comments
16			
17			
18			
19			
20			
21			
22			
23			
24			
25			
26			
27			
28			
29			
30			

Walking Your Way To Better Health

Don't ignore your holistic self - care because you are walking 10,000 steps a day

Don't ignore your holistic self-care because you are walking 10,000 steps a day. You also have to stay vigilant during your daily activities and interactions with others. Stay vigilant when talking to others. Understand that differences in opinion, differences in perception of reality, differences in emotional reaction to similar situations and circumstances or even how things can be done, can lead to escalation of negativity. How can walking help you to manage the escalation of negativity in your daily interactions with others? Even a 20-minute walk will help you lift your mood and clear your head.

Walking Your Way To Better Health

Remember that "Your present circumstances don't determine where you can go; they merely determine where you start." Nido Qubein. Remember that a positive mindset can help you find hope even in the most challenging situations and circumstances.

Research has shown that those with a growth mindset make positivity the unifying motivational thread throughout all these changes that they deal with every day. Focus more on finding positive solutions in every encounter than on complaining.

Don't let others discourage you from going for your walk every day. Remember that maintaining a daily walking routine is part of the telomeric lifestyle. Check yourself and make you are sticking to walking at least 10,000 steps every day. A combination of exercise, eating healthy and managing stress with good self-care will help you live a healthy and long life in a realistic and sustainable way.

What are the positive adjustments you can make every day? Don't try to please everyone. Stop complaining and focus on what you can control.

What steps do you need to take every day to help with improving your holistic self-care as you continue to walk towards better health? How many adjustments did you make in the past 7 days that helped you diffuse tension and get more of the positive results you wanted in your daily activities and interactions with others? Don't forget to make seeing your doctor or your provider part of your journey to better health.

Remember that to foresee is to rule. Form the habit of looking at things, situations and even the achieving of your goals from a solutions perspective rather than from a blaming and complaining perspective. A situation that requires a solution can be approached in a variety of ways. Expect the unexpected.

Do you know the most common factors that can affect your holistic self-care? Do your own 72-hour audit to get an idea. Some of the factors that can affect your holistic self-care would include the falls and accidents already mentioned above and other factors that include personal habits and community relationships.

Don't focus so much on walking at least 10,000 steps, that ignore near and immediate health challenges like falls , accidents or unexpected health conditions.

Drink a lot of water when the weather is hot to avoid getting dehydrated and falling. Don't drive too fast. What if you had started your morning with your morning exercise and meditation but because you were running late to work or a meeting you forgot to put on your seat belt, and while driving too fast ended up in an accident? Will this be a good outcome for your better health or longer life? What was going on in your mind?

Don't ignore unexpected health conditions. Don't ignore or dismiss nagging or persistent symptoms without proper checkup because this could be the difference between discovering cancer at an early stage or at an advanced stage.

Keep an eye on yourself through the regular use of health and wellness journals or even the appendix in this book that contains the compass profile and other tables, trackers and journals that you can fill up as part of holding yours.

Don't ignore going for your yearly physical or doing your recommended screening tests because of your age or family circumstance or history because you are busy or don't really feel like it.

*Have you reviewed your health insurance in the past 30 days?

*Do you put in the time to learn more about the things that are good for your health?

*Do you say 3 things you are grateful for every day?

How many times did you fall or have a near fall in the past 7 days? Keep a close eye on your physical environment and stay vigilant with your health and self-care in the next 30 days, starting from today.

Walking Your Way To Better Health

Walking every day can help improve your whole-body health

Research shows that a sedentary lifestyle is considered a significant risk factor for cardiovascular disease while consistently doing more physical activity could be considered a non-pharmacological intervention for improving cardiovascular fitness in healthy and diseased individuals. Increase daily physical activity improves quality of life, reduces body weight, reduces LDL cholesterol, increases HDL cholesterol, increases insulin sensitivity, and helps to prevent pathologic conditions like obesity, atherosclerosis, diabetes, and decreases blood pressure both at rest and during exercise, thus preventing a hypertensive state (Sorriento, Vaia and Iaccarino, 2021)

Walking regularly is one of the easiest ways to improve your health from head to toe. According to the Cleveland clinic regular exercise can make a significant difference in improving how your body and brain function. Research shows that walking can improve your brain health.

According to the NIH, studies show that exercise can improve cognitive function through neurophysiological changes. Research found that regular exercise such as walking every day can help to induce positive changes in the brain, like improved neurogenesis and angiogenesis and upregulated neurotrophic factors possibly leading to increased neurons and neuronal networks (Kang et al, 2021). Exercise will help you to counter the decline in neurons and neuronal networks that typically occurs as you get older.

Remind yourself that you are trying to protect your brain health and preserve your cognitive functions such as attention, learning, thinking, problem solving, decision making, and memory for as long as you can as you get older. The more you preserve your cognitive functions and memory as you get older, the less mistakes, accidents and falls you are likely to have as you get older.

One thing you can do that will help protect your brain health and memory will be taking more steps every day and possibly doing more puzzles or doing more activity books weekly. How well are you keeping up with doing 10,000 steps a day? Check your responses to the tables in this book or go to the 30 -day walking challenge tracking part of this book to hold yourself accountable.

Research has shown that walking helps boost your mood because it increases blood flow and blood circulation to the brain and body. Researchers at New Mexico Highlands University (NMHU) found that the foot's impact during walking sends pressure waves through the arteries that significantly modify and can increase the supply of blood to the brain. Please don't tell me you are too stressed out to walk. You are too stressed out not to walk. Walking will help you melt away stress and keep your organs younger!

Walking Your Way To Better Health

Did you know that forming the habit of doing more physical activity is one of the keys to living longer? Did you know that research shows that not exercising increases your risk of premature death more than cardiovascular disease, diabetes and even smoking? Interestingly, according to Bringham Young University researchers, exercise has antiaging effects at the cellular level because increasing physical activity increased the length of telomeres at the end of chromosomes which are usually shorter with age. The study also found that those who exercise had a "biological age" that was about nine years younger(Baines, 2020; Crouch 2019).

Research has shown that people as old as 69 years and above who exercise regularly have the heart, lung, and muscle fitness of healthy people as young as 30 years and younger(Crouch, 2019). Are you beginning to see that walking every day can help to improve your whole-body health?

Your hobbies could be playing baseball, basketball, golf, dancing, fishing, running,

Walking Your Way To Better Health

Do you have a family or personal history of obesity–related illnesses like diabetes, high blood pressure, heart attack or stroke? If you have a blood pressure cuff, measure your blood pressure today. If you do not have one, go to the nearest pharmacy, and use their free blood pressure cuff to find out your blood pressure. Do you know that walking every day can help you deal with these health challenges?

How does physical activity affect your cellular and vascular health? As you already know, consistent physical activity helps to increase the length of your telomeres at the cellular level. At the vascular level , exercise protects the endothelium or cells lining the vessels by reducing reactive oxygen species and reducing inflammation by increasing the synthesis of anti-inflammatory cytokines or chemicals and increases the cellular metabolic state by increasing mitochondrial biogenesis and autophagic influx (Sorriento, Vaia and Iaccarino, 2021). Mitochondria are critical to human health and in organs in which damaged mitochondria accumulate more organ damage or disorders occur(Sorriento, Vaia and Iaccarino, 2021).

Do you know that walking can also help improve your eye health? Do you want to see better as you get older? Walk more. According to American Ophthalmology Association research suggests that moderate physical activity can help people with diabetes reduce the risk of eye diabetic retinopathy and other eye problems that can cause of loss of vision among working age adults. Don't forget that walking at least 10,000 steps a day is an example of moderate physical activity that can help you keep up with the CDC recommended physical activity level of at least 30 minutes a day, since walking 10,000 steps a day is equal to about 100 minutes of exercise.

How else does physical activity help your eyes? Research shows that if you already have an eye disease, exercise may help you manage it better and people who engaged in moderate physical exercise were less likely than inactive people to develop glaucoma.

According to the Cleveland clinic research shows that two and a half to five hours of moderate intensity exercise per week — which includes walking — can help reduce your risk of certain cancers like colon, breast, endometrial, kidney, liver, multiple myeloma and non-Hodgkin lymphoma. You already know that walking at least 10,000 steps a day will help double your two and half hours of moderate intensity exercise to at least 8 hours of exercise per week. After all, waking 10,000 steps per day is about 100 minutes of physical activity per day, when you do that for at least 5 days a week, it becomes about 500 minutes a week, which is at least 8 hours of physical activity per week.

You have to be more intentional and decisive as you get older. Research has shown that if you were exercising when you were younger then stopped exercising as you got older, you would increase your risk of having a deadly stroke. On the other hand, if you started exercising between 40 and 60 years, you would reduce your risk of having stroke that can significantly reduce your chances of living longer. This shows that it is really never too late to start exercising or form the habit of consistently increasing the level of your physical activity.

Do you know that walking every day can help to protect your joints? According to the Cleveland clinic walking can help to strengthen your muscles and increase blood flow to your cartilage. This can be especially helpful if you are dealing with joint pain or arthritis. I know this counter intuitive, but walking is a low- impact exercise that can help to keep your joints flexible and reduce the risk of osteoporosis.

Do not think that it is either you are getting everything right or everything is wrong. If you plan to walk 100 minutes a day but due to circumstances beyond your control you were able to do only 50 minutes, you have not failed. Do the 50 minutes that day, then do 150 minutes the next day to make it up. This makes a total of 200 minutes in two days. On the third day you can go back to 100 minutes a day. Be flexible but make sure you are also tracking your progress.

Walking Your Way To Better Health

How many steps do you take every day? What are you waiting for?

According to the CDC an estimated 110,000 deaths per year could be avoided if US adults 40 years and older increased their moderate-to vigorous exercise by even as little 10 minutes more a day. The question you need to ask is "Can you find 10 more minutes in your busy daily schedule to do more physical activity?" What is holding you back from walking your way to good health? Is it time? Are you too busy or too distracted? How many steps per day have you taken in the last 7 days? How minutes of walking did you do yesterday ? Was it up to 100 minutes? Make sure you walk at least 10,000 steps a day in walking your way to better health compass challenge.

Remember to make sure you are paying attention to managing active-illness and potential long-term problems

What is your self-care strategy for managing active illness? Don't assume that because you are walking every-day, that you don't have to collaborate with your doctors to make sure that everything that you need to take care of health wise is being done.

If you have not seen your doctor in a long time set up an appointment with your health care provider so that you can get a more detailed picture of your metabolic profile, especially your cholesterol level, blood sugar, potassium, vitamin D and other tests relevant to your family and medical history.

What are the other important self-care aspects you need to know and do. Do you brush your teeth every morning and night?

Do you ignore your oral health and personal hygiene in your health and wellness journey? **Poor oral health can lead to systemic diseases like heart disease, pneumonia and cancer to name a few.**

Don't forget your eyes. Do you see your eye doctor regularly? Do you know that research shows that taking 5 mg of melatonin every night can help your eye health? Do you know that research shows that walking about 60 minutes a day for about five times a week can help to lower your intraocular pressure (IOP) and improve blood flow to the brain and the eye (Schmidt KG et al, 1996)? Research shows that walking about 5,000 steps a day can help to decrease visual field loss in glaucoma patients.

When was the last time you saw your doctor? Do you get your immunizations as needed? If you need to get vaccines, get your vaccines like the flu vaccines or COVID 19 vaccines. Do not just say you are eating healthy, exercising, and taking your supplements; therefore, you do not need to get your vaccines. If you need to bundle up because it is cold, do it. Wash your hands frequently to minimize your chances of getting an infection.

Do you also know that focusing on gratitude despite your daily changes can be part of your daily self-care?

What about sociocultural self-care? Are you a value adding person? Do you add value to your culture and community? As you get older people can say that you have contributed positively to your cultural heritage. Do you stay connected to your community?

What about your spiritual self-care? Do what is right for your spirituality without condemning others? Do you do your meditation and regularly go to your faith-based services? Research shows that if you have a lifestyle with spirituality and religion, you have a healthier and longer life!

What is holding you back from improving your health every day? Is it that you are too busy? Is it that you don't have a better self-mastery of yourself? While self-mastery requires more mental energy to set up, once you have achieved greater self-mastery you will require less energy to function more effectively through good positive healthy habits.

Do you deal with stress by smoking or drinking alcohol? Do you know that drinking too much alcohol is not good for your health?

*Don't smoke. If you are still smoking, make plans to stop. Don't use smoking, alcohol and sex as coping mechanisms for managing stress or dealing with challenging or negative relationships.

Consider taking advantage of free informational health exams or blood work offered at your office or your membership clubs or insurance to get your cholesterol or metabolic profile.

*Do you have a family history of high blood pressure, diabetes, cancer, or glaucoma?

Walking Your Way To Better Health

*Start each day with meditation and exercise and a plan for the day. Make this part of your compass blueprint or process.

*Keep quiet if you have nothing positive to say.

*Become familiar with your family and medical history.

*Review your health insurance regularly.

*Get more the education that will help you become a better health self-advocate

*Stay vigilant in all your interactions with others.

* What area of self -improvement did you focus on in the past 72 hours?

*Forgive yourself and others daily

*Sleep at least seven to eight hours a day.

Walking Your Way To Better Health

*Cut down on unnecessary expenses.

*Call a friend today.

*Review your finances monthly

*How much money do you make in a week and how much money do you spend in a week?

*Help at least one person each day.

*Meditate or say a prayer or do both.

*Form a healthy living group of friends and family that you can trust or join one.

*Check your blood pressure weekly.

*Weigh yourself weekly

*Take your multivitamins regularly.

*Do you protect your home from falls and accidents?

Walking Your Way To Better Health

*Do you work for your future every day or do you get easily distracted and postpone everything to tomorrow?

.

*Do you write down your emotional challenges every 3 days?

*Work for your future everyday

.*Continue to write on journal at least once a week.

.

After the check up, you have to follow through with the labs and tests you have to do. You have to go to the pharmacy and get your medications. After you get your medications, you must take them or make sure you don't mix them up when taking them, if not you will not get the desired result.

Please write down how many times you took your medications in the past 7 days. Use your 30-day tabulation or journal notes, to keep yourself accountable, starting from today. The point is that walking your way to better health does not occur in isolation. You must include a holistic approach that involves other aspects or part of your life.

Review what you have done and challenge yourself to use your holistic habits for walking to better health

One of the habits that can help you achieve better health is working 10,000 steps per day. While consistently walking 10,000 steps over the next 30 days and beyond will help you to improve your health, it will not happen in a vacuum. You may have to start with as low as 2000 steps per day then build up. You may also have to support your daily walking with holistic habits.

A habit can be defined or described as a behavior that is recurrent, that is acquired or formed through repeated action that is usually brought on by a cue or social context (Rubin, 2015).

Walking Your Way To Better Health

Challenge yourself to form habits that will help you review and improve daily. What is the essence of your walking every day if it will not help you live a happy, healthy, longer, and more positive and fulfilled life? Are you intentional enough or do you get easily distracted?

Your brain likes to reduce the energy it uses to accomplish tasks, which is part of the reason we form habits. Research has shown that about 40 % to 50% of our daily activities are shaped by habits. Do you know the habits that dominate your own daily activities? Are they good habits or bad habits? Have you formed the habit of walking at very least 5,000 steps every day and avoiding daily distractions?

Start each day with your 12 Compass walking your way to better health guidelines. Here are examples of the few things you can do regularly as part of daily holistic self-care:

*Start each day with meditation, exercise and a to-do list

Walking Your Way To Better Health

*Sleep at least seven to eight hours a day

*How many times did you reach out to a friend or relative in the past one week?

 *What simple steps can you take today to have better health?

*Do you meditate every day?

Have you formed a healthy living group of friends and family that you can trust or joined one that can help you stick to walking 10,000 steps a day? Remember that consistency is the key to getting the health benefits of waking your way to better health.

*How many hours a day do you spend on social media or on the phone?

*Get a blood pressure logbook and use it.

*Keep your appointment with your healthcare providers.

Walking Your Way To Better Health

 *When was the last time you did your yearly physical?

*Take care of your oral health, personal hygiene and self-care

*Do you do your screening tests as recommended by your healthcare providers?
*Become familiar with your family and medical history.

*Have you reviewed your health insurance in the past 30 days?

*Do you put in the time to learn more about the things that are good for your health?

*Do you say 3 things you are grateful for every day?

*How many hours do you spend watching TV every day? Is it distracting you from walking your daily steps?

*How many steps did you take today? Do you know that you can use walking to cope

with stress or deal with your daily challenges?

Start your own walking journal with some of the answers to the above questions and related guidance. Start a health and wellness journal. Get pen and paper and write down your own answers to the questions above or type them into your computer, phone, or mobile device. Do some journaling to help you hold yourself more accountable.

Keeping to the 80:20 rule through your habits, daily activities, and lifestyle changes will help begin to live a healthier, happier, longer and more fulfilled life as you continue to walk 10,000 steps every day.

In order to become more consistent with walking 10,000 steps a day, do the 30-day walking your way to better health challenge that looks at how many steps you take every day, your motivation for walking, and how would manage your situation and circumstance better. You can also write down your concerns on the time of walking (morning, afternoon or night), distractions you dealt with), and hours of sleep. The goal is to hold yourself accountable and find the blueprint that would help you to be more consistently effective. Don't forget to look at your compass profile and the appendix at the end of this book!

DAY 1 of 30-day walking your way to better health challenge.

Table of number of steps and minutes of walking

Day	Number Of Steps	Minutes of walking	Day	Number Of Steps	Minutes Of walking
1			16		
2			17		
3			18		
4			19		
5			20		
6			21		
7			22		
8			23		
9			24		
10			25		
11			26		
12			27		
13			28		
14			29		
15			30		

Comments and Concerns:

Make   more notes. Did you do your 10,000 steps today? Make notes on what motivated you to   do your 10,000 steps today or on what prevented you from doing your 10,000 steps today. How will you handle   your situation and circumstances going forward?

DAY 2 of 30-day walking your way to better health challenge.

Table of number of steps and minutes of walking

Day	Number Of Steps	Minutes of walking	Day	Number Of Steps	Minutes Of walking
1			16		
2			17		
3			18		
4			19		
5			20		
6			21		
7			22		
8			23		
9			24		
10			25		
11			26		
12			27		
13			28		
14			29		
15			30		

Comments and Concerns:

Make   more notes. Did you do your 10,000 steps today? Make notes on what motivated you to do your 10,000 steps today or on what prevented you from doing your 10,000 steps today. How will you handle your situation and circumstances going forward?

DAY 3 of 30-day walking your way to better health challenge.

Table of number of steps and minutes of walking

Day	Number Of Steps	Minutes of walking	Day	Number Of Steps	Minutes Of walking
1			16		
2			17		
3			18		
4			19		
5			20		
6			21		
7			22		
8			23		
9			24		
10			25		
11			26		
12			27		
13			28		
14			29		
15			30		

Comments and Concerns:

Make   more notes. Did you do your 10,000 steps today? Make notes on what motivated you to do your 10,000 steps today or on what prevented you from doing your 10,000 steps today. How will you handle your situation and circumstances going forward?

DAY 4 of 30-day walking your way to better health challenge.

Table of number of steps and minutes of walking

Day	Number Of Steps	Minutes of walking	Day	Number Of Steps	Minutes Of walking
1			16		
2			17		
3			18		
4			19		
5			20		
6			21		
7			22		
8			23		
9			24		
10			25		
11			26		
12			27		
13			28		
14			29		
15			30		

Comments and Concerns:

Make   more notes. Did you do your 10,000 steps today? Make notes on what motivated you to do your 10,000 steps today or on what prevented you from doing your 10,000 steps today. How will you handle your situation and circumstances going forward?

DAY 5 of 30-day walking your way to better health challenge.

Table of number of steps and minutes of walking

Day	Number Of Steps	Minutes of walking	Day	Number Of Steps	Minutes Of walking
1			16		
2			17		
3			18		
4			19		
5			20		
6			21		
7			22		
8			23		
9			24		
10			25		
11			26		
12			27		
13			28		
14			29		
15			30		

Comments and Concerns:

Make   more notes. Did you do your 10,000 steps today? Make notes on what motivated you to do your 10,000 steps today or on what prevented you from doing your 10,000 steps today. How will you handle your situation and circumstances ?

DAY 6 of 30-day walking your way to better health challenge.

Table of number of steps and minutes of walking

Day	Number Of Steps	Minutes of walking	Day	Number Of Steps	Minutes Of walking
1			16		
2			17		
3			18		
4			19		
5			20		
6			21		
7			22		
8			23		
9			24		
10			25		
11			26		
12			27		
13			28		
14			29		
15			30		

Comments and Concerns:

Walking Your Way To Better Health

Make   more notes. Did you do your 10,000 steps today? Make notes on what motivated you to do your 10,000 steps today or on what prevented you from doing your 10,000 steps today. How will you handle your situation and circumstances ?

DAY 7 of 30-day walking your way to better health challenge.

Table of number of steps and minutes of walking

Day	Number Of Steps	Minutes of walking	Day	Number Of Steps	Minutes Of walking
1			16		
2			17		
3			18		
4			19		
5			20		
6			21		
7			22		
8			23		
9			24		
10			25		
11			26		
12			27		
13			28		
14			29		
15			30		

Comments and Concerns:

Make   more notes. Did you do your 10,000 steps today? Make notes on what motivated you to do your 10,000 steps today or on what prevented you from doing your 10,000 steps today. How will you handle your situation and circumstances ?

DAY 8 of 30-day walking your way to better health challenge.

Table of number of steps and minutes of walking

Day	Number Of Steps	Minutes of walking	Day	Number Of Steps	Minutes Of walking
1			16		
2			17		
3			18		
4			19		
5			20		
6			21		
7			22		
8			23		
9			24		
10			25		
11			26		
12			27		
13			28		
14			29		
15			30		

Comments and Concerns:

Make   more notes. Did you do your 10,000 steps today? Make notes on what motivated you to do your 10,000 steps today or on what prevented you from doing your 10,000 steps today. How will you handle your situation and circumstances ?

DAY 9 of 30-day walking your way to better health challenge.

Table of number of steps and minutes of walking

Day	Number Of Steps	Minutes of walking	Day	Number Of Steps	Minutes Of walking
1			16		
2			17		
3			18		
4			19		
5			20		
6			21		
7			22		
8			23		
9			24		
10			25		
11			26		
12			27		
13			28		
14			29		
15			30		

Comments and Concerns:

Make   more notes. Did you do your 10,000 steps today? Make notes on what motivated you to   do your 10,000 steps today or on what prevented you from doing your 10,000 steps today. How will you handle your situation and circumstances ?

DAY 10 of 30-day walking your way to better health challenge.

Table of number of steps and minutes of walking

Day	Number Of Steps	Minutes of walking	Day	Number Of Steps	Minutes Of walking
1			16		
2			17		
3			18		
4			19		
5			20		
6			21		
7			22		
8			23		
9			24		
10			25		
11			26		
12			27		
13			28		
14			29		
15			30		

Comments and Concerns:

Make   more notes. Did you do your 10,000 steps today? Make notes on what motivated you to do your 10,000 steps today or on what prevented you from doing your 10,000 steps today. How will you handle your situation and circumstances ?

DAY 11 of 30-day walking your way to better health challenge.

Table of number of steps and minutes of walking

Day	Number Of Steps	Minutes of walking	Day	Number Of Steps	Minutes Of walking
1			16		
2			17		
3			18		
4			19		
5			20		
6			21		
7			22		
8			23		
9			24		
10			25		
11			26		
12			27		
13			28		
14			29		
15			30		

Comments and Concerns:

Make   more notes. Did you do your 10,000 steps today? Make notes on what motivated you to do your 10,000 steps today or on what prevented you from doing your 10,000 steps today. How will you handle your situation and circumstances ?

DAY 12 of 30-day walking your way to better health challenge.

Table of number of steps and minutes of walking

Day	Number Of Steps	Minutes of walking	Day	Number Of Steps	Minutes Of walking
1			16		
2			17		
3			18		
4			19		
5			20		
6			21		
7			22		
8			23		
9			24		
10			25		
11			26		
12			27		
13			28		
14			29		
15			30		

Comments and Concerns:

Make   more notes. Did you do your 10,000 steps today? Make notes on what motivated you to do your 10,000 steps today or on what prevented you from doing your 10,000 steps today. How will you handle your situation and circumstances ?

DAY 13 of 30-day walking your way to better health challenge.

Table of number of steps and minutes of walking

Day	Number Of Steps	Minutes of walking	Day	Number Of Steps	Minutes Of walking
1			16		
2			17		
3			18		
4			19		
5			20		
6			21		
7			22		
8			23		
9			24		
10			25		
11			26		
12			27		
13			28		
14			29		
15			30		

Comments and Concerns:

Make   more notes. Did you do your 10,000 steps today? Make notes on what motivated you to do your 10,000 steps today or on what prevented you from doing your 10,000 steps today. How will you handle your situation and circumstances ?

Walking Your Way To Better Health

DAY 14 of 30-day walking your way to better health challenge.
Table of number of steps and minutes of walking

Day	Number Of Steps	Minutes of walking	Day	Number Of Steps	Minutes Of walking
1			16		
2			17		
3			18		
4			19		
5			20		
6			21		
7			22		
8			23		
9			24		
10			25		
11			26		
12			27		
13			28		
14			29		
15			30		

Comments and Concerns:

Make   more notes. Did you do your 10,000 steps today? Make notes on what motivated you to do your 10,000 steps today or on what prevented you from doing your 10,000 steps today. How will you handle your situation and circumstances going forward?

DAY 15 of 30-day walking your way to better health challenge.

Table of number of steps and minutes of walking

Day	Number Of Steps	Minutes of walking	Day	Number Of Steps	Minutes Of walking
1			16		
2			17		
3			18		
4			19		
5			20		
6			21		
7			22		
8			23		
9			24		
10			25		
11			26		
12			27		
13			28		
14			29		
15			30		

Comments and Concerns:

Make   more notes. Did you do your 10,000 steps today? Make notes on what motivated you to do your 10,000 steps today or on what prevented you from doing your 10,000 steps today. How will you handle your situation and circumstances ?

DAY 16 of 30-day walking your way to better health challenge.

Table of number of steps and minutes of walking

Day	Number Of Steps	Minutes of walking	Day	Number Of Steps	Minutes Of walking
1			16		
2			17		
3			18		
4			19		
5			20		
6			21		
7			22		
8			23		
9			24		
10			25		
11			26		
12			27		
13			28		
14			29		
15			30		

Comments and Concerns:

Walking Your Way To Better Health

Make   more notes. Did you do your 10,000 steps today? Make notes on what motivated you to   do your 10,000 steps today or on what prevented you from doing your 10,000 steps today. How will you handle your situation and circumstances ?

DAY 17 of 30-day walking your way to better health challenge.

Table of number of steps and minutes of walking

Day	Number Of Steps	Minutes of walking	Day	Number Of Steps	Minutes Of walking
1			16		
2			17		
3			18		
4			19		
5			20		
6			21		
7			22		
8			23		
9			24		
10			25		
11			26		
12			27		
13			28		
14			29		
15			30		

Comments and Concerns:

Make   more notes. Did you do your 10,000 steps today? Make notes on what motivated you to do your 10,000 steps today or on what prevented you from doing your 10,000 steps today. How will you handle your situation and circumstances ?

DAY 18 of 30-day walking your way to better health challenge.

Table of number of steps and minutes of walking

Day	Number Of Steps	Minutes of walking	Day	Number Of Steps	Minutes Of walking
1			16		
2			17		
3			18		
4			19		
5			20		
6			21		
7			22		
8			23		
9			24		
10			25		
11			26		
12			27		
13			28		
14			29		
15			30		

Comments and Concerns:

Make   more notes. Did you do your 10,000 steps today? Make notes on what motivated you to do your 10,000 steps today or on what prevented you from doing your 10,000 steps today. How will you handle your situation and circumstances ?

DAY 19 of 30-day walking your way to better health challenge.

Table of number of steps and minutes of walking

Day	Number Of Steps	Minutes of walking	Day	Number Of Steps	Minutes Of walking
1			16		
2			17		
3			18		
4			19		
5			20		
6			21		
7			22		
8			23		
9			24		
10			25		
11			26		
12			27		
13			28		
14			29		
15			30		

Comments and Concerns:

Make   more notes. Did you do your 10,000 steps today? Make notes on what motivated you to do your 10,000 steps today or on what prevented you from doing your 10,000 steps today. How will you handle your situation and circumstances ?

DAY 20 of 30-day walking your way to better health challenge.

Table of number of steps and minutes of walking

Day	Number Of Steps	Minutes of walking	Day	Number Of Steps	Minutes Of walking
1			16		
2			17		
3			18		
4			19		
5			20		
6			21		
7			22		
8			23		
9			24		
10			25		
11			26		
12			27		
13			28		
14			29		
15			30		

Comments and Concerns:

Make   more notes. Did you do your 10,000 steps today? Make notes on what motivated you to do your 10,000 steps today or on what prevented you from doing your 10,000 steps today. How will you handle your situation and circumstances ?

DAY 21 of 30-day walking your way to better health challenge.

Table of number of steps and minutes of walking

Day	Number Of Steps	Minutes of walking	Day	Number Of Steps	Minutes Of walking
1			16		
2			17		
3			18		
4			19		
5			20		
6			21		
7			22		
8			23		
9			24		
10			25		
11			26		
12			27		
13			28		
14			29		
15			30		

Comments and Concerns:

Make   more notes. Did you do your 10,000 steps today? Make notes on what motivated you to do your 10,000 steps today or on what prevented you from doing your 10,000 steps today. How will you handle your situation and circumstances ?

DAY 22 of 30-day walking your way to better health challenge.

Table of number of steps and minutes of walking

Day	Number Of Steps	Minutes of walking	Day	Number Of Steps	Minutes Of walking
1			16		
2			17		
3			18		
4			19		
5			20		
6			21		
7			22		
8			23		
9			24		
10			25		
11			26		
12			27		
13			28		
14			29		
15			30		

Comments and Concerns:

Make   more notes. Did you do your 10,000 steps today? Make notes on what motivated you to do your 10,000 steps today or on what prevented you from doing your 10,000 steps today. How will you handle your situation and circumstances ?

DAY 23 of 30-day walking your way to better health challenge.

Table of number of steps and minutes of walking

Day	Number Of Steps	Minutes of walking	Day	Number Of Steps	Minutes Of walking
1			16		
2			17		
3			18		
4			19		
5			20		
6			21		
7			22		
8			23		
9			24		
10			25		
11			26		
12			27		
13			28		
14			29		
15			30		

Comments and Concerns:

Walking Your Way To Better Health

Make   more notes. Did you do your 10,000 steps today? Make notes on what motivated you to do your 10,000 steps today or on what prevented you from doing your 10,000 steps today. How will you handle your situation and circumstances ?

DAY 24 of 30-day walking your way to better health challenge.

Table of number of steps and minutes of walking

Day	Number Of Steps	Minutes of walking	Day	Number Of Steps	Minutes Of walking
1			16		
2			17		
3			18		
4			19		
5			20		
6			21		
7			22		
8			23		
9			24		
10			25		
11			26		
12			27		
13			28		
14			29		
15			30		

Comments and Concerns:

Walking Your Way To Better Health

Make   more notes. Did you do your 10,000 steps today? Make notes on what motivated you to do your 10,000 steps today or on what prevented you from doing your 10,000 steps today. How will you handle your situation and circumstances ?

DAY 25 of 30-day walking your way to better health challenge.

Table of number of steps and minutes of walking

Day	Number Of Steps	Minutes of walking	Day	Number Of Steps	Minutes Of walking
1			16		
2			17		
3			18		
4			19		
5			20		
6			21		
7			22		
8			23		
9			24		
10			25		
11			26		
12			27		
13			28		
14			29		
15			30		

Comments and Concerns:

Make   more notes. Did you do your 10,000 steps today? Make notes on what motivated you to do your 10,000 steps today or on what prevented you from doing your 10,000 steps today. How will you handle your situation and circumstances ?

DAY 26 of 30-day walking your way to better health challenge.

Table of number of steps and minutes of walking

Day	Number Of Steps	Minutes of walking	Day	Number Of Steps	Minutes Of walking
1			16		
2			17		
3			18		
4			19		
5			20		
6			21		
7			22		
8			23		
9			24		
10			25		
11			26		
12			27		
13			28		
14			29		
15			30		

Comments and Concerns:

Make   more notes. Did you do your 10,000 steps today? Make notes on what motivated you to do your 10,000 steps today or on what prevented you from doing your 10,000 steps today. How will you handle your situation and circumstances ?

DAY 27 of 30-day walking your way to better health challenge.

Table of number of steps and minutes of walking

Day	Number Of Steps	Minutes of walking	Day	Number Of Steps	Minutes Of walking
1			16		
2			17		
3			18		
4			19		
5			20		
6			21		
7			22		
8			23		
9			24		
10			25		
11			26		
12			27		
13			28		
14			29		
15			30		

Comments and Concerns:

Make   more notes. Did you do your 10,000 steps today? Make notes on what motivated you to do your 10,000 steps today or on what prevented you from doing your 10,000 steps today. How will you handle your situation and circumstances ?

DAY 28 of 30-day walking your way to better health challenge.

Table of number of steps and minutes of walking

Day	Number Of Steps	Minutes of walking	Day	Number Of Steps	Minutes Of walking
1			16		
2			17		
3			18		
4			19		
5			20		
6			21		
7			22		
8			23		
9			24		
10			25		
11			26		
12			27		
13			28		
14			29		
15			30		

Comments and Concerns:

Walking Your Way To Better Health

Make   more notes. Did you do your 10,000 steps today? Make notes on what motivated you to   do your 10,000 steps today or on what prevented   you from doing your 10,000 steps today. How will you handle your situation and circumstances ?

DAY 29 of 30-day walking your way to better health challenge.

Table of number of steps and minutes of walking

Day	Number Of Steps	Minutes of walking	Day	Number Of Steps	Minutes Of walking
1			16		
2			17		
3			18		
4			19		
5			20		
6			21		
7			22		
8			23		
9			24		
10			25		
11			26		
12			27		
13			28		
14			29		
15			30		

Comments and Concerns:

Make   more notes. Did you do your 10,000 steps today? Make notes on what motivated you to do your 10,000 steps today or on what prevented you from doing your 10,000 steps today. How will you handle your situation and circumstances ?

DAY 30 of 30-day walking your way to better health challenge.

Table of number of steps and minutes of walking

Day	Number Of Steps	Minutes of walking	Day	Number Of Steps	Minutes Of walking
1			16		
2			17		
3			18		
4			19		
5			20		
6			21		
7			22		
8			23		
9			24		
10			25		
11			26		
12			27		
13			28		
14			29		
15			30		

Comments and Concerns:

Make   more notes. Did you do your 10,000 steps today? Make notes on what motivated you to do your 10,000 steps today or on what prevented you from doing your 10,000 steps today. How will you handle your situation and circumstances ?

Walking Your Way To Better Health

Appendix I : The compass profile

What is the Compass Profile? Do you know how the different components of the compass profile can help you do better?

The components of the compass profile are the following:

C=	Community	Relationships	or Communication profile.
O = Operational capacity profile.
M= Metabolic profile.
P= Physical profile.
A= Ambition profile.
S= Spiritual profile.
S = Self Knowledge profile.

The COMAPASS METHOD is the holistic approach to continuous self-improvement and transformation in health, wellness, and self-mastery based on using the compass profiles and specific compass guidelines.

Understanding and applying the different compass profiles to your situation and circumstances will help you become better at dealing with the root cause of the factors affecting your health and your ability to become a better version of yourself.

The community relationships profile is essentially your communications profile. The way you communicate and relate with yourself and with others will affect whether you will have value- adding relationships or not. Do you know what is affecting your confidence in yourself and your ability to make effective decisions? Is it fear of the process or fear of communication with others? Is it fear of failure? Communicate with yourself first and write down your deepest fears and worries. Is it what others will say?

Ask yourself questions that will help you recognize which aspects of your relationship with others could either be contributing to your failure to build positive and supportive relationships or could be making things worse. Remember that when you are communicating with others, they will interact with you from their own perspective, worldview, personality, or experience.

Lower your expectations that others will understand you or see things from your perspective. Don't let others frustrate you or disrupt your focus on meeting your 30 -day challenge for living longer.

What is your operational capacity profile? Your operational capacity is your ability to get things done or to make adjustments when the going gets tough and still get things done. Minimize excuses and explanations. The key is that you need to know your limitations or challenges and how to navigate through them. What resources do you have to support or help you as you continue to try to do the specific 30-day compass challenge that you have to do?

Do you know how to look at problems as gifts, and challenges as opportunities? Try to reduce complex problems to small segments that you can accomplish. Begin where you are, not where you want to be. Step by step do the possible.

Do you know your metabolic profile? This is a way of looking at yourself at the micro level or microenvironment. When was the last time you got your blood work done? Your **metabolic profile** will include both your nutritional and metabolic analysis. You can get your metabolic analysis by getting your appropriate physiological and laboratory tests done. help. Getting the right tests done with the help of a healthcare professional or your doctor will make it easy for you to know which aspect of your health you need to focus on improving.

The Physical Profile includes your weight, height, waist circumference, BMI (Body Mass Index) and your environment. It also includes your heart rate and lung function. Movement and structures in your body are a big part of your physical profile. Make sure you exercise every day in a safe environment so that avoid falls and exposure to avoidable harm. Keep it simple and moderate , if you want something more vigorous check with your doctor before you begin. After all, checking with your doctor or getting additional information from an expert is a very important part of self-care.

The fifth compass profile is your ambition profile. You can use your ambition profile to assess your drive and motivation. What motivates you? What are your goals? Are you motivated more by the thoughts of success, or fear of failure? You can use the ambition profile to s**et measurable goals like walking at least 10,000 steps a day or eating at least 50 g of fiber every day.** Are you motivated enough to achieve your goals through determination and commitment? **Don't quit at the first obstacle.**

The remaining two profiles are **Spirituality and Self Knowledge profiles. The compass spirituality profile focuses on your** relationship with yourself, others, your community, the universe or with God, if you are a person of faith. Do you have a sense of connection to a higher power or does a purpose beyond yourself or your own benefits drive your thoughts, meditations, and actions? How can you apply your own spiritual profile to the 30-day compass longevity challenge? A better understanding of your sense of self will help you develop your own positive warrior mindset in a way that will work for you.

The seventh compass profile is your self-knowledge life. Do you know if you have predominantly positive thinking or negative thinking? Do you know your **personality,** personality traits or tendencies, character and mindset? Do you have self-mastery?

A better understanding of your psychosocial strengths and weaknesses will help you know your limitations, and your tendencies, when it comes to forming holistic habits and taking simple steps that will help you live a healthier and longer life.

You can use the 7 components of the compass profile to develop a more holistic approach to living a healthier and longer life.

Appendix II: Tables, trackers and journals

TABLE 1A

Day	Number Of Steps	Minutes of walking	Motivation For walking	Reason For Not Walking	comment
1					
2					
3					
4					
5					
6					
7					
8					
9					
10					
11					
12					
13					
14					
15					

TABLE 1B

Day	Number Of Steps	Minutes of walking	Motivation For walking	Reason For Not Walking	comment
16					
17					
18					
19					
20					
21					
22					
23					
24					
25					
26					
27					
28					
29					
30					

Walking Your Way To Better Health

TABLE 2A

Day	Number Of Steps	Minutes of walking	Number of distractions
1			
2			
3			
4			
5			
6			
7			
8			
9			
10			
11			
12			
13			
14			
15			

Walking Your Way To Better Health

TABLE 2B

Day	Number Of Steps	Minutes of walking	Number of distractions
16			
17			
18			
19			
20			
21			
22			
23			
24			
25			
26			
27			
28			
29			
30			

Walking Your Way To Better Health

TABLE 3 A

Day	Number Of Steps	Minutes of walking	Motivation For walking	How many distractions did you overcome	comment
1					
2					
3					
4					
5					
6					
7					
8					
9					
10					
11					
12					
13					
14					
15					

Walking Your Way To Better Health

TABLE 3 B

Day	Number Of Steps	Minutes of walking	Motivation For walking	How many distractions did you overcome	comment
16					
17					
18					
19					
20					
21					
22					
23					
24					
25					
26					
27					
28					
29					
30					

Walking Your Way To Better Health

TABLE 4A

Day	Number Of Steps	Hours on TV	Number of Distractions	Hours of Sleep
1				
2				
3				
4				
5				
6				
7				
8				
9				
10				
11				
12				
13				
14				
15				

Walking Your Way To Better Health

TABLE 4B

Day	Number Of Steps	Hours on TV	Number of Distractions	Hours of Sleep
16				
17				
18				
19				
20				
21				
22				
23				
24				
25				
26				
27				
28				
29				
30				

Walking Your Way To Better Health

TABLE 5A

Day	Blood Pressure	weight	Number of daily steps	Comments
1				
2				
3				
4				
5				
6				
7				
8				
9				
10				
11				
12				
13				
14				
15				

Walking Your Way To Better Health

TABLE 5B

Day	Blood Pressure	weight	Number of daily steps	Comments
16				
17				
18				
19				
20				
21				
22				
23				
24				
25				
26				
27				
28				
29				
30				

Walking Your Way To Better Health

TABLE 6A

Day	Number Of Steps	weight	Blood pressure	Number of out bursts of stress
1				
2				
3				
4				
5				
6				
7				
8				
9				
10				
11				
12				
13				
14				
15				

TABLE 6B

Day	Number Of Steps	weight	Blood Pressure	Number of out bursts of stress
16				
17				
18				
19				
20				
21				
22				
23				
24				
25				
26				
27				
28				
29				
30				

Walking Your Way To Better Health

SIMPLE WEIGHT TRACKER

DATE	TIME	WEIGHT	NOTES / COMMENTS

TABLE 7A

Day	Number Of Steps	Compass Stress index (CSI)	comments
1			
2			
3			
4			
5			
6			
7			
8			
9			
10			
11			
12			
13			
14			
15			

Walking Your Way To Better Health

TABLE 7B

Day	Number Of Steps	Compass Stress Index(CSI)	comments
16			
17			
18			
19			
20			
21			
22			
23			
24			
25			
26			
27			
28			
29			
30			

Walking Your Way To Better Health

12 COMPASS WALKING YOUR WAY TO BETTER HEALTH GUIDELINES

Do you?	1	2	3	4	5	6	7	8	9	10
Meditate on 3 things you are grateful for daily										
Do 10,000 steps daily										
Sleep At Least 7 hours A Day										
Walk at least 50 minutes every day										
Do daily self-accountability										
Effectively manage daily stress										
Lower daily expectations										
Maintain a healthy weight										
Keep your health vigilance										
Have Supportive relationships										
Eat five servings of vegetables and fruit daily										
Write 3 good things that happened to you every day										

Notes

Ardell DB(1999), Definition of wellness. Ardell Wellness Report,1999, 1-5.

Bains P (2020) Exercise to live longer. Allina Health

Be well BU; Learn practices that lead to better   health   and   well-being. www.belmont.edu

Bussing A, Wirth AG, Reiser F, Zahn A, Humbroich K, Gerbersghagen K, Baumann K. Experience of gratitude, awe and beauty in life among patients with multiple sclerosis and psychiatric disorders. Health Qual Life outcomes.2014;12:63. https://pubmed.ncbi.nim.nih.gov/25102199/

CDC.gov; LDL and HDL Cholesterol: "Bad" and "Good" Cholesterol

Crouch M(2019) AARP

Chung I, (2005)Stress-Induced Atherosclerosis: Clinical Evidence and Possible Underlying Mechanism, Korean Circulation J 2005;35:101-105
Microsoft Word - 순2-1.doc (koreamed.org)

Debbie L Stoewen, (2017) Dimensions of Wellness. Can Vet J, 58(8): 861-862

Healing yourself with self-hypnosis, Frank Caprio, M.D. and joseph R Berger

Kang SJ, Kim BH, Lee H, Wang J. The Beneficial Effects of Cognitive Walking Program on Improving Cognitive Function and Physical Fitness in Older Adults. Healthcare (Basel). 2021 Apr 5;9(4):419. doi: 10.3390/healthcare9040419. PMID: 33916351; PMCID: PMC8066196.

Lin, J. and Epel, E.(2022) Stress and telomere shortening; Insights from cellular mechanisms. Ageing Res Rev.2022

Jan:73:101507. Published online 2021 Nov 1.doi 10.1016/j.arr.2021.101507

Mels Carbonell, Ph.D., How to solve the people puzzle. Uniquely You Resources, 2008.

Mills PJ, Redwine L, Wilson K, Pung MA, Chinh K, Greenberg BH, Lunde O, Maisel A, Raisinghani A, Wood A, Chopra D. The Role of Gratitude in Spiritual Well-being in Asymptomatic Heart Failure Patients. Spiritual Clin Pract (Wash D C). 2015 Mar;2(1):5-17. doi: 10.1037/scp0000050. PMID: 26203459; PMCID: PMC4507265.

National Council on Aging(NCOA).(2023), Get the facts on Healthy Aging. www.ncoa.org

National Institutes of Health(.gov) https://www.ncbi.nih.gov.pmc
NSC(National Safety Council)2023: Injury Facts: Deaths by Demographics: Top 10 Preventable Injuries
https://injuryfacts.nsc.org//all-in

National Institute of Health(NIH) News.(2017), You're Never too Old. Keep active as you age. https;//newsinhealth.nih.gov/special-issues/seniors/youre-never-too-old

Poljšak B, Milisav I. Clinical implications of cellular stress responses. Bosn J Basic Med Sci. 2012 May;12(2):122-6. doi: 10.17305/bjbms.2012.2510. PMID: 22642596; PMCID: PMC4362434

Robin G. Better Than Before: Mastering the Habits of Our Everyday Lives.Toronto, Ontario, Pengium Random House, Doubleday Canada, 2015.

Renna, M.E.(2021) A review and novel theoretical model of how negative emotions influence inflammation: The critical role of emotion regulation. Brain Behav Immun Health. 2021,Nov 25. Doi:10.1016/j.bbih.2021.100397 Retrieved from https://www.ncbi.nlm.nih.gov/pmc/articles/PMC8649080/

Sabot D, Lovegrove R, Stapleton P. The association between sleep quality and telomere length: A systematic literature review. Brain Behav Immun Health. 2023 Jan 9;28:100577. doi: 10.1016/j.bbih.2022.100577. PMID: 36691437; PMCID: PMC9860369.

Salleh MR. Life event, stress and illness. Malays J Med Sci. 2008 Oct;15(4):9-18. PMID: 22589633; PMCID: PMC3341916.

Schmidt KG et al. *Graefes Arch Clin Exp Ophthalmol.* 1996;234(8):527-532.

Shammas MA. Telomeres, lifestyle, cancer, and aging. Curr Opin Clin Nutr Metab Care. 2011 Jan;14(1):28-34. doi: 10.1097/MCO.0b013e32834121b1. PMID: 21102320; PMCID: PMC3370421.
Sorriento D, Di Vaia E, Iaccarino G. Physical Exercise: A Novel Tool to Protect Mitochondrial Health. Front Physiol. 2021 Apr 27;12:660068. doi: 10.3389/fphys.2021.660068. PMID: 33986694; PMCID: PMC8110831.

Smith, K. S., & Graybiel, A. M. (2016). Habit formation. *Dialogues in clinical neuroscience, 18*(1), 33–43. https://doi.org/10.31887/DCNS.2016.18.1/k smith
Retrieved from Habit formation (nih.gov)

University of New Hamshire2023, Health & Wellness. www.unh.edu
https://www.unh.edu/health/intellectual wellness
University of Maryland:Dimensions of Wellness. Retrieved from (last accessed 2021)
https://www.umaryland.edu/wellness/dimen sions-of-wellness

Wood AM, Maltby J. Stewart N, Linley PA, Joseph S.(2008). A social-cognitive model of trait and state levels of gratitude. Emotion,2008;8(2):281-280.
https://pubmed.ncbi.nim.nih.gov   [Google Scholar]

WHO (2020)The top ten causes of death

Walking Your Way To Better Health

https://www.who.int/news-room/fact-sheets/details/the-top-10-causes-of-death

Yaribeygi H, Panahi Y, Sahraei H, Johnston TP, Sahebkar A. The impact of stress on body function: A review. EXCLI J. 2017 Jul 21;16:1057-1072. doi: 10.17179/excli2017-480. PMID: 28900385; PMCID: PMC5579396.

Walking Your Way To Better Health

Resources

Here are additional resources that will help you live a healthier and longer life by consistently trying to be the best version of yourself in all aspects of your life. Did you know that you can become the best and happiest version of yourself every day irrespective of the situation or circumstance you may find yourself in?

www.compasswellnessinstitute.com

http://www.amazon.com/Dr.-Chio-Ugochukwu/e/B00JNFLPQQ

Join the compass club on Facebook

https://www.facebook.com/groups/1748276835431116/

Other books by Dr. Chio Ugochukwu that will help you improve your health, eliminate stress and transform your life include;

The Compass Health Transformer: Your 72 Hour Blue Print For Healthy Living

In this book you will learn more about how doing the 72-hour food audit can help you gain a better understanding of how you can improve your health through easy daily adjustments …..

21 Ways To Transform Your Health Without Medications

"…21 simple proven ways to reduce stress and improve your health and wellbeing without relying on medications. These are easy and effective ways you can use to turn your daily challenges into transformative opportunities for healthy living and daily happiness. You can start right away without spending a fortune!.."

<u>Get your own copy of 21 Ways To Transform Your Health Without Medications</u>

Overcoming Daily Stress: 21 Quick And Easy Ways To Stay Stress-Free In Your Daily Life

"…Are you tired of being stressed out everyday? Are you tired of feeling exhausted and overwhelmed in your daily activities? Are you fed up with communication issues in your relationship? Here are 21 quick and easy ways you can use to overcome daily stress and turn your daily challenges into opportunities for transformative abundant living. This book will help you gain a better understanding of your potential communication issues, daily 'stress points' and the steps you can take to overcome them…".

Get your own copy of Overcoming Daily Stress

The Secret To Daily happiness

"..Have you ever wondered why daily happiness has continued to elude you? Do you want to make sustainable daily happiness part of your life? By reading this book
you can find answers to these questions and many more on how to overcome the many obstacles and challenges that daily try to take away your inner peace and contentment…"

<u>Get your own copy of The Secret To Happiness</u>

15 Simple Ways to lower your blood pressure naturally after 40 without complicated diets

"……Don't spend your most productive years dealing with high blood pressure, medications and side effects. Stop worrying about whether you forgot to take your first medication or the second one. Take these simple steps to lower your blood pressure naturally and minimize your need for multiple medications. Did you know that high blood pressure can cause heart attacks, stroke, kidney failure, blindness and memory problems? Don't wait to find out! Take Action! ,,,,,"

<u>Click Here for Your own copy of 15 Simple Ways To Reduce Blood Pressure....</u>

Here is a book to help lose fat. If your main concern or focus is losing pounds you have accumulated as fat then get a copy of the book

Walking Your Way To Better Health

"How To Lose 23 Pounds of Fat Without Torture Diets or Hard Exercise And keep it (The Compass Method).

"Are you fed up with trying to lose weight again and again with limited success? Are you tired of all the confusing new and expensive diets you have tried to follow every day with zero results? Do you want the health benefits of living with optimum weight without following complicated rules? Do you want to become more energetic and active again? Are you fed up with the wild ride of losing weight today and gaining it back tomorrow? Then read this book so that you will start using a comprehensive individualized weight loss strategy that will help you lose fat and keep it off, without going on torture diets or deadly strenuous exercises. You will learn to do this through the Compass Method that is based on a holistic approach to weight-loss, healthy living and personal transformation."

If prayer is something that appeals to you, you might be interested in the following next two books that incorporate prayers into our daily strive to become better and become more fulfilled:

Praying To Win: How To Get More Victories And Riches In Your Daily Life Through Spiritual Principles

"..You too can achieve your goals and dreams, through praying to win. You can do this by immersing yourself in the word of God and transforming the moments that make up your daily life through persistent adoration……. Above all, thank God every day, never give up and persistently continue praying to win…"

Get your own copy of Praying To Win

9 Best Ways To Eliminate Stress, Improve Your Health And thrive Without Limitations Through Prayers

Are tired of being knocked down by stress from your daily hassles? Are you tired of dealing with chronic illnesses associated with stress? Do you want to live a fun-filled daily life? Here are 9 of the best ways you can change your daily obstacles and challenges into opportunities to thrive without limitations through the power of prayers.

Too Young To Die

"A book about coping with grief and finding your way in life…"

9 Best Ways To Quit Smoking Without Becoming A Nervous Wreck And Gaining Weight

"..Here are 9 of the best ways to finally quit smoking without becoming a nervous wreck or gaining weight. If you have tried to quit smoking before, but failed or tried to quit but was overcome by anxiety or fear of becoming socially awkward or gaining weight, then read this book! This book was previously published as "The Compass Health Transformer Quit Smoking" but has been rewritten to include the transtheoretical model of change to help you get a better understanding of where you are in your journey or process of quitting smoking. The

9 best ways to quit smoking also includes a reminder of the different ways smoking can affect your health and body and the different individualized-changes you can make to your life-style to help you quit smoking on your own terms.

9 Best Ways To Deal With Negative People, Protect Your Health And Be Happy

"..Are you tired of being stressed out by encounters with negative people? Are you fed up with the impact of negative situations on your health and happiness? Would like you to find out ways to remain effective during negative situations and encounters with negative people? Do you know that chronic stress generated by negative encounters can damage your eyes, heart and brain? Do you know that chronic stress can directly damage your body cells? Here are 9 best ways you can protect your health from such negative situations so that you can continue to thrive and be happy..".

Walking Your Way To Better Health

To order new or additional copies or ask questions, please visit:

http://www.amazon.com/Dr.-Chio-Ugochukwu/e/B00JNFLPQQ

Call or Text : 661 992 6436

Join the Compass club @

https://www.facebook.com/compassclub

Walking Your Way To Better Health

About the Author

Dr. Chio Ugochukwu has always been interested in helping people live healthier, longer and more fulfilled lives through daily improvements in their health and wellness, and better self-care. He is focused on helping individuals and groups, use the compass method to develop their own compass blueprint or process for healthy living, and self-mastery. Doing the 30-day challenge in this book will help you have better health and live longer by learning how to stay more consistently physically active, improve your self-accountability and health vigilance, sleep better, become more efficient at managing stress, and chronic conditions, and have more positive and supportive relationships.

Dr. Chio was inspired to develop the compass method for transformational living, through the challenges he has encountered in his journey of life, his practice of medicine, and his fascination with how the mind, the spirit and human experience influence the accomplishment of goals and the fulfillment of life, and his ancient heritage of Ozaa Akwusina (Warriors Never Stop).

He is the medical director of the Compass Wellness Institute and a consultant and specialist with interests in integrative medicine, ophthalmology, medical informatics, and public health. As an author, researcher, and consultant, he has peer reviewed publications on health and quality of life, and published more than 100 books and articles, on health and wellness, eye health, weight management, conflict management, stress management, effective communication, and integrative self-mastery.

To get some of Dr. Chio's books please visit:
https://www.amazon.com/author/chio